Lamby

A Mother's Journey Through a Twisted

Medical System to Save Her Son

Nikki Polidori

For Carrie, my other half, and Pickle – my hero!

Prologue

My son was due at Christmastime. What better omen could there have been that he would be a happy, healthy child who would bring endless joy to our lives?

The truth is that he *does* bring endless joy, but the path from where we started to where we are now has not been an easy one. Instead of a child whose only tears would be shed over a misplaced pacifier, my son's first few years have been challenging ones that have forced both of us to fight for his life and taught me that we're both far stronger than we might appear to be.

Thursday, December 8, 2005

The baby is coming two weeks early! I was in the kitchen when my water broke. Matt was there, along with a friend, sitting around the counter and talking about how much money they'll make if Connecticut gets the 6-to-12-inch snowfall that's predicted. I'll admit that this snowplowing side business has been lucrative, and it's fun for them.

Bella (our Westie) needed to go out; and, as I stood outside with her, that familiar smell of an upcoming snow was in the air. Apparently, the weather forecasters were right this time. The night was dark, so Bella wasn't distracted by the shadows she sees on brighter nights. She did her business quickly, and we headed back inside. I sat down on a stool at the counter, and she plopped down at my feet. She kept nudging my leg, asking to be petted. They say dogs have instincts, so I guess she was trying to tell me something.

I was flipping through a catalog when my water broke. I quietly excused myself and snuck upstairs. By the time I got there, my pants were soaked! Immediately, my mind went back two years to Sydney's birth. I'd been taking a walk with Mom when my water broke. Since I had no contractions, I took my time; and we arrived at the hospital just six hours before our beautiful little girl was born.

When I got back downstairs, I was wearing clean pants and a smile. Matt gave me a quizzical look, asking why I had changed. I was impressed that he noticed and said "It's time to go".

In a matter of seconds, our friend was gone; and Matt and I were left to take care of a few things before leaving for the hospital. I called my doctor, who advised us to leave right away to avoid any chances of the baby being born on the highway in the middle of a snowstorm; but I knew we had plenty of time. I went into my home office to complete some last-minute work. Matt decided to take a nap. When Sydney was born, he was exhausted after being up all night.

By the time I'd finished my work, I was having cramps that were gradually increasing in strength; but I wasn't concerned. I looked in on Sydney, who was sleeping soundly, and smiled at how her life was about to change with the birth of her baby brother. I took a shower and packed my bag.

As my contractions amped up, I called Mom, who arrived within minutes, to take care of Sydney. By now, I was becoming pretty uncomfortable and anxious to get going. Matt? Not so much. It took me ten minutes to get him up from his nap. Then, we had the debate over which car to take for the 45 minute trip to the hospital. I wanted the wagon. Matt insisted on the truck, since it has four-wheel drive, oblivious to the fact that it would be a pretty bouncy ride, not to mention hard for me to climb into the seat. But, – whatever.

Friday, December 9, 2005, 10:00 a.m.

What a night! It was midnight by the time we got to the hospital. I changed into my fabulous hospital gown, feeling pretty much like a whale at this point. Then, I listened to the baby's heartbeat on the monitor and waited for my epidural. I'd only dilated to 3 cm, but my contractions were pretty brutal. I really needed that epidural, and it was taking forever! I couldn't help thinking that we weren't getting off to the best start.

It took four attempts – four very *painful* attempts – to get the epidural in place. I'm no expert, but I'd been through this before. I can't help but wonder if the anesthesiologist knew what he was doing (after all, this *is* a "teaching" hospital). By the time he was finally in, I hardly noticed that I was in labor because the pressure in my spine took over everything. I never moved or even screamed, but it's entirely possible that I broke the nurse's fingers. I'll never forget her face.

Finally, I was able to lie back and try to get some rest before delivery time. My OB, Dr. Randall, had come and gone; and it was just Matt and me in the room. I was just starting to drift off when machines started beeping all around me. Instantly, a crowd of people came rushing into the room. A nurse leaned over me and said, "Don't try to get up. *DO NOT MOVE!*" Comforting, right? Then, Dr. Randall came rushing in. So much for his usual quiet demeanor. He reassured me, though, that the baby would be fine.

At this point, I think there were three doctors and two nurses hovering over me, giving me something through my IV and watching the monitor to see if the numbers would change. Apparently, my blood pressure had dropped to 42/17, which was clearly a bad situation. I felt a little dizzy, but I'm not sure if it was from the bottomed-out BP or just from the panic I was starting to feel because of all the activity. With Sydney, I'd been left alone forever between checks; and there were times when I wondered if they expected me to deliver the baby myself. Not so this time! I don't know what set everything off; but, after an hour or so – plus three shots of epinephrine – my BP was back to normal, and I was told to rest. Easier said than done.

After a while, a nurse came in. I told her I was feeling a lot of pressure very low. When she checked, all of a sudden my bed got ripped apart. I found myself sitting up, trying to help the nurse move my legs into the stirrups. You know what? It's hard to get your feet into those things when you have no feeling in them! The nurse alerted Matt just as Dr. Randall came in and told me to start pushing. We were on our way.

My almost-8-pound baby boy was born at 5:20 a.m. He's so cute! He has dark hair and dark eyes to match. He even looks like he has a tan. He's going to be a heartbreaker! We're naming him Dylan.

Friday, December 9, 2005, 8:00 p.m.

After last night's frantic activity, I've been alone almost all day. After I moved to the post-partum unit, Matt went home to spend time with Sydney and to give my mom a chance to come and meet her new grandson. It's been nice to have some time alone with Dylan; but it's been a little stressful, too. I don't remember Sydney spitting up this much, and I'm sure she didn't choke like Dylan does. Every time I hear these strange noises, I grab him and hold him upright; but I'm not sure it's helping much. I asked the nurse about it, and she said that sometimes when babies are born quickly like Dylan was they swallow a bit of mucus; and this is how they clear it out of their system. I guess that makes sense, but it's a little disconcerting.

He's a cutie, though!

Saturday, December 10, 2005

I think there's something wrong with Dylan.

The nurses keep insisting that he's fine and still trying to get rid of all the gunk he ingested during the birth process, but I don't think all this coughing is normal. It's not really a typical cough – more of a loud, deep barking sound that reminds me of a seal. Surely, that can't be right. It makes me a little nervous about leaving the hospital. Everyone says he's okay, and I guess they know best; but I also trust my own instincts as a mother. It just doesn't seem right to me. We're seeing the pediatrician in three days, so I guess I'll bring it up then. In the meantime, Dylan and I are going home! I'm excited to start life with our expanded family and enjoy the best Christmas yet.

Friday, December 16, 2005

Whew! No time to write with the craziness of having a newborn and a two year old, plus the pre-holiday craziness. We've been going through the typical newborn stuff – no sleep, constant feedings, never-ending laundry and bottles to be washed, cooking, playing with Sydney, and attending to Dylan. Occasionally, I even get to take a shower! We're settling into a comfortable routine now, and life is good.

I'm still worried about the barking, though. When Dylan coughs, and sometimes after he eats, he makes that seal-like sound that just doesn't seem right. Feeding him isn't easy either. Sydney was such a good eater from the very beginning, but not so with him. Instead of falling asleep after a feeding, he gets really fussy. He doesn't want to lie on his back. If I pick him up, he quiets down immediately and falls asleep. The problem is that when I put him back down he starts fussing again. Obviously, I can't sit up all night and hold him while he sleeps, so I've got to figure something out.

Saturday, December 17, 2005

We got a little bit of relief last night. I talked to a couple of seasoned moms, and they recommended letting him sleep in his car seat so that he'd be a little more upright. It helped a little. He's been sleeping about two hours before he wakes up and starts to fuss again; but he's starting to get congested, too, especially at night. I guess every baby is different, but I know we didn't have these issues with Sydney. Maybe we just got spoiled!

Friday, December 23, 2005

Well, the car seat solution was nice while it lasted; but now it's stopped working. I took him to the doctor today to see what's going on. The pediatrician, Dr. Mateo, said that he has a cold and that's what is causing the nasal congestion. I don't know how a two-week-old would get a cold, since he hasn't been around anyone who's sick. But, ok. He said to run a humidifier and try to get him to sleep on his side. Let's hope that works.

Tuesday, December 27, 2005

I'm so exhausted that I can barely move. Dylan's sleeping hasn't improved at all. After I feed him, the only way he'll sleep is if I hold him upright on top of me; but, of course, the pediatrician lectured me about that. Really, though. What am I supposed to do? He's got to get some rest somehow. And so do I.

Thursday, December 29, 2005

I've found a potential solution to the sleeping arrangements. I sit partially upright with a big pillow wedged under each armpit. Then, I lay Dylan on my chest, put a baby blanket across his back, and tuck the ends under me. I figure this way, if he rolls over, at least he'll stay in place and won't get crushed or dropped. I'm sure it looks pretty ridiculous, but at least he's sleeping a few hours at a time; and I'm getting a little more rest. His cold hasn't gone away, though; and now he's started spitting up, which causes him to choke. It's pretty scary sometimes. I think I'll try laying him on his side, so he won't choke. Maybe if I put some rolled towels in the bassinet, it will hold him in place so that he won't roll over.

Friday, December 30, 2005

New problem – diarrhea! Can you believe it? This isn't the normal loose stools that a lot of newborns have. I'm talking about pure liquid that comes in amazing fluorescent colors.

This started two days ago, and we were getting eight of these bizarre stools a day; so off to the pediatrician we went. This time we saw Dr. Colbert, who said Dylan has some kind of viral infection and that there's nothing to be done but wait for it to pass in a few days. This baby is having the worst luck ever! But, hopefully, all of this will turn around in the New Year.

Friday, January 6, 2006

Another trip to Dr. Mateo today. The choking episodes are getting worse and worse, and it just doesn't seem right to me.

If I was expecting a sympathetic ear and a solution, I was pretty far off base. Dr. Mateo wasn't sure what to make of my complaints. I told him that the coughing and choking really had me concerned, but he acted like I was just one of those new mothers who worry needlessly about everything. He just kind of shrugged it off.

However, he did have a solution to offer for the sleeping problems. He told me to let Dylan "fuss it out." Um . . . I'm not one to coddle a baby unnecessarily, and I do think there are certain situations in which you should let a baby cry a bit; but this just doesn't seem like one of them.

I don't know what to think. Am I being paranoid or worried for no reason? I don't think so. I'm a new mom, but I'm not a first-time mom. I've been through the whole newborn thing with Sydney, and we didn't have *anything* like the issues we're having with Dylan. I know I need to trust the doctors. They've got degrees and plenty of experience, so they should know what they're doing; but I also trust my own instincts and education. I think there's more to it than a cold or a spoiled baby, who should just cry it out.

Thursday, January 12, 2006

Another week, another trip to the doctor. I don't think Sydney went this often in her first six months!

I decided to switch pediatricians. Today, we saw Dr. Barclay. I went through his entire history with her – the congestion, the frequent choking, the barking when he coughs, the sleeping problems, and the diarrhea that's lasted two weeks now. I also mentioned that his breathing sounds wet sometimes. She diagnosed him with acid reflux disease and started him on Prevacid, which she thinks will help a lot.

She was less sure about the diarrhea. She agreed with Dr. Colbert (initial pediatrician) that it's probably a viral thing and said we should just keep an eye on it.

The good news is that, despite all these issues, Dylan is gaining weight and looks great; so Dr. Barclay doesn't think there's cause for alarm. We'll see.

Thursday, January 19, 2006

Well, Dr. Barclay said to take Dylan *off* the Prevacid that we just started a week ago because it might be causing his diarrhea. Aaaggghhhh.

Tuesday, January 24, 2006

Last night was SCARY. All of us had gone to bed, and we'd been asleep for a while, when Dylan started choking so badly that he couldn't breathe. I was panic-stricken and nearly called the paramedics, but then he got over it. I thought he was okay.

I went back to bed but had trouble sleeping, which turned out to be a good thing. The baby monitor was cranked up to the highest volume, and I thought I heard Dylan cry once. It was faint. There was a pause that all my instincts said was lasting too long, and then the coughing started again. I think I learned to fly at that point, because I was in his room almost instantly. The poor little guy was choking and having trouble breathing again, and he was soaked from the vomit in his crib. After he calmed down and I got him cleaned up, I put him back to bed with his new favorite toy, a flat lamby with soft fur on one side and silk on the other. I went back to bed, but there was no more sleeping for me. All I did was lie awake and listen to the monitor.

First thing this morning, I called Dr. Barclay's office. They said she was on vacation. Of course she is, because nothing has been easy since this baby was born! They referred me to the on-call doctor; and he agreed to see us this afternoon, thank God. He didn't have any answers but gave me a referral to Dr. Feinstein, who is a pediatric ear, nose, and throat specialist. He's going to work us in quickly.

Wednesday, January 25, 2006

Saw Dr. Feinstein (ENT) today. Finally, we might have an answer. He says Dylan has something called laryngomalacia, which is exacerbated by his reflux. Apparently, it's a pretty rare condition that occurs when the soft cartilage in a baby's larynx collapses inward when he inhales, which obstructs his airway. This condition also causes something called stridor, which Dr. Feinstein says is the source of the wheezing sounds that have had me so worried and could also be causing his feeding problems.

This all sounds very, very scary to me; but the doctor doesn't seem to be worried. He says the condition usually resolves itself in time. He did tell me to watch Dylan carefully and to let him know immediately if he ever turns blue. WHAT? You can bet I'll call someone immediately if my little guy turns blue!

He told us to start the Prevacid again (after starting it two weeks ago and stopping it one week ago . . .), but give it to him 15 or 20 minutes before he eats. He gave us another appointment in three weeks. In the meantime, I'm trying to relax a little more, knowing that I'm not a crazy, paranoid new mom. These things are NOT just in my imagination. They're real, and there's an explanation – even a name for it; and time should take care of the situation. I did some Internet research that confirmed everything Dr. Feinstein said, so I do feel better, although I'm still on guard. Knowing he might turn blue makes me want to never take my eyes off him!

Thursday, January 26, 2006

Back to Dr. Barclay's (pediatrician) office today. I told her he STILL has diarrhea – nearly six weeks now. She took him off his regular formula and started him on Alimentum, which is supposed to be better for food allergies and colic.

Tuesday, February 14, 2006

Dylan and I took a little field trip today – to the pediatric ER in New Haven – just to get a "fresh, independent opinion". He's been on the Alimentum formula for two weeks now. There's been no change at all, plus his breathing is getting more noisy; and he's been really, really irritable.

What a waste of time! They put down that he had diarrhea and colic, and I guess it's their policy to check in with the child's pediatrician. They called Dr. Barclay. Okay, that's fine; but, instead of backing me up and noting Dylan's ongoing issues, she showed up, took over with no new thoughts or treatment offered by anyone at all and essentially kicked us out of the ER. I couldn't believe it. Her discharge note said, "I'm not sure why she came to the ER – apparently the baby was extremely fussy today" and that she'd handle it. If she had been "handling it", I wouldn't have had to go to the ER in the first place! And, Dylan is way beyond "fussy." The poor kid has had chronic diarrhea and this weird choking thing since he was born. He must be miserable, and God knows I am.

I'm not too impressed with Dr. Barclay right now, but she did say she'd consult with a pediatric gastroenterologist and get back to me.

Oh, and one other thing. The hospital put Dylan's gender down as "female." A real confidence builder.

Wednesday, February 15, 2006

Dr. Barclay called me back today. She's spoken with Dr. Boyer, the pediatric gastroenterologist that she mentioned yesterday. It looks like we're changing formulas again. This doctor wants Dylan to try something called Neocate, which she says is good for babies who have various kinds of gastric problems; and he definitely does! I also need to call her office for an appointment. I'm losing track of the number of doctors Dylan has seen in his short life, but I'm determined to keep going until we get the right answers.

Monday, February 20, 2006

The night chokings are occurring almost every night now. Some episodes are worse than others, but it's safe to say that no one is getting much sleep around here.

Take last night, for example. When Dylan has a choking incident, he usually pulls out of it within 30 seconds to a minute, which seems like a lifetime when it's happening. But, last night it went on for several minutes. I was getting really scared, so I took Dylan into our bedroom. I turned on the bedroom light to see if Dylan was turning blue. I couldn't quite tell about his skin color.

I was getting frantic and was about to call 911, but then he got better, thank God. Once he got calmed down (and I did, too – at least a little), I changed him and put him back to bed with Lamby. Then, I slept in his room the rest of the night. Well, I didn't sleep so much as cried most of the night, for a LOT of reasons. I'm physically and emotionally exhausted, desperately worried about Dylan, and increasingly convinced that I'm in this by myself. Nights like this, I could use a lamby of my own.

Wednesday, March 8, 2006

We finally saw Dr. Boyer (pediatric GI) today. She didn't spend a lot of time examining him, but she said pretty quickly that he has severe reflux and increased his Prevacid to 30 mg. She wants to see him again, when he hits the 6-month mark, to check on his progress and re-evaluate things. She said we should start to see improvement in the spitting up and irritability. Hope she's right!

Thursday, March 9, 2006

Looks like there will be no vacation for me. It seems like forever since we've gone on a trip (unless you count driving to Dylan's various doctors' offices), so I've been REALLY looking forward to going to Florida with Mom, Sydney, Dylan and my cousin, aunt, and nephew. Matt didn't want to go because he's planned a ski trip out West with his buddies.

But, it looks like we're not going anywhere. Dylan has had a low-grade fever for five days and just hasn't looked well all week. Dr. Barclay (pediatrician) thinks we should cancel the trip. She's afraid the change might make him worse, and she's probably right. No sense taking a chance on a vacation with a sick baby. That wouldn't be all that much fun, but I'm still disappointed.

Needless to say, Matt's plans didn't change. He's off to the slopes while I stay home with the kids.

Saturday, March 11, 2006

I might not be in Florida, but I did take a trip today – to the mall. Today's shopping trip was partly for fun but mostly a necessity. Dylan's constant spitting up has ruined many of my clothes. Now he's on a formula called Neocate; and, besides having to take out a second mortgage to pay for it, it smells horrible and stains worse than tomato sauce. In the past few weeks, I've thrown out five pairs of pants and more than a dozen shirts because they've been stained beyond repair. So much for wearing my cute clothes again, now that I'm not pregnant anymore! Thank God, no one sees me when I'm at home, because I've started to wear shirts that are already stained, rather than take a chance on ruining more clothes. So, now I have a few new things. I'll save them for when I go out and just hope they survive!

My wardrobe isn't the only thing that's taking a beating. The only way Dylan is comfortable is if you're holding him upright. Whether we're at home or out somewhere, he's always upright and over my shoulder. Then, without warning, there's what I call a "silent explosion," followed by a loud splat when the vomit hits the floor. This kid defines the term "projectile vomiting." It can literally land five feet behind my shoulder. I can't imagine that we're very popular when we go out.

Sunday, March 12, 2006

No improvement so far, since starting the new formula and increasing the Prevacid. In fact, the spitting up is more severe and happening more often than ever. Frustrating!

Wednesday, March 15, 2006

Okay. This is getting ridiculous. Dylan spit up 26 times yesterday. Yep. I kept a log.

I keep thinking about when Sydney was this age. Feeding her was such a joy! She'd look into my eyes and touch my hand as I'd hold the bottle, and I felt this overwhelming sense of love.

What a difference this time around. I dread feeding time; and I guess Dylan does, too. As soon as I start giving him the bottle, he starts crying. Then, the choking starts. He's got to be hungry; but, for some reason, eating is a really unpleasant experience for him and, frankly, for me, too. I worry about him because he refuses to eat for days at a time. Feeding him has turned into a scientific process, rather than the pleasurable experience it should be. Instead of the peaceful feeling I had when I fed Sydney, now I feel frustrated and upset; and so does Dylan. I love this little guy so much. My heart breaks for him because something is clearly wrong, and I don't know what to do to fix it.

I thought I'd get some help from Dr. Boyer (GI); but, when I called the office, they told me to just deal with it. I thought she'd want to see him. But no. I guess we'll keep plugging away.

Monday, March 20, 2006

Again, something new! Dylan is still spitting up 20 or 30 times a day EVERY DAY, but today his "offering" contained something that looked like coffee grounds. What can THAT be??? I called Dr. Barclay (pediatrician), who told me it was Malory-Weiss Syndrome.

I looked it up, and the dictionary said it is bleeding from tears in the mucosa at the junction of the stomach and the esophagus and is usually caused by severe retching, coughing, or vomiting. It's a condition that's commonly associated with alcoholism or eating disorders like bulimia. We don't have any of that, but we certainly have coughing and vomiting in spades.

When we got home, I called Dr. Boyer (GI). She wouldn't give him an appointment but did prescribe by phone something called Reglan. Before getting the prescription filled, I did some research. That is a BAD DRUG! The list of side effects include dyskinesia, seizures, rapid heart rate . . . it went on and on. No way am I giving anything like that to my kid.

Friday, March 31, 2006

Saw Dr. Barclay (pediatrician) today for what was technically Dylan's four-month check-up. But, it's not like we've been strangers to her office. I've lost track of how many times I've been there in the past few weeks. I've talked with her extensively about his difficulty eating, noisy breathing, irritability, refusal to take his bottle, and the continued vomiting – including the fact that he's still spitting up the "coffee grounds" several times a day. All she ever says is that "reflux can be bad sometimes." No kidding!

I'm at my wits end. Does she think I'm imagining things? Or, that I'm exaggerating? Or, that I'm a bad mother? She seems so unconcerned, but I'm with this little guy 24 hours a day. I KNOW something is not right, but I don't feel like anyone is listening to me.

Monday, April 10, 2006, 9:00 a.m.

The last few days have been a whirlwind, but now we are at the hospital and waiting for Dylan to come back from an upper GI endoscopy. I absolutely hate the idea of our tiny son going under anesthesia and having a tube stuck down his throat. But, I'm also very grateful that Dr. Boyer finally decided to do something. Hopefully, this procedure will give us the answers we're looking for. I am holding Lamby for Dylan while he's having his endoscopy. I hope it will be a small piece of comfort for him as he's waking up. And, to be honest, it's a comfort for me right now, too.

Monday, April 10, 2006, 6:30 p.m.

Finally home. What a nightmare. Dr. Boyer (GI) came out after the procedure and said she'd found a "pretty good-sized" S-curve in Dylan's esophagus, which she thinks is a hiatal hernia. She also said she saw no evidence of reflux. So, why have we been treating him for it all this time?? Aaagghh.

We were happy when the procedure was over, but then we saw Dylan. He looked . . . I can't even describe it. His breathing was soooo noisy, and he was bucking and squirming all over the place. We couldn't get a bottle into him without him choking. I held him and rocked him, thinking maybe I could comfort him and calm him down; but he was beyond uncomfortable, and the bucking just wouldn't stop. Nothing I did seemed to help much, so we were both pretty frustrated and unhappy.

We thought we were ready to go home at that point, but they decided to keep him a couple of extra hours for observation because of something that happened in the OR that caused them to give him a vapo-nebulizer of epinephrine. I asked for more information, but no one seemed to know anything more. Poor little guy is exhausted, and so am I.

Thursday, April 13, 2006

Today, we had to see Dr. Barclay (pediatrician). The past few days have been horrible – respiratory distress; wet breathing. He is obviously uncomfortable, and there's nothing we can do about it. He's 4 months old but sometimes breathes like an old man with emphysema. Dr. Barclay didn't have anything new to offer. She suggested we see Dr. Feinstein (ENT) again, which we'll do tomorrow.

In the meantime, I might have found a new source for information and help. I went to the dentist today; and, when the receptionist asked about the kids, I laid out everything we've been going through and how distressed I am about all of it. I wouldn't have told all that to a stranger, but she's an old family friend; and I found myself pouring my heart out to her. I went to grade school with her daughter Samantha and had forgotten that she is now a pediatric cardiologist at a children's medical center in Pennsylvania. She gave me Samantha's e-mail address and suggested that I see if she has any thoughts, so I sent her a note tonight. I haven't seen her in years, but I do know her well and felt comfortable contacting her. And, let's face it. I'd reach out to just about anyone at this point.

Friday, April 14, 2006

Dr. Feinstein (ENT) didn't have any answers either, so he called Dr. Boyer (GI) to find out more about the endoscopy. Turns out Dylan had a desaturation episode in the OR while he was intubated. This means his oxygen level dropped significantly, as did his blood pressure, which is why they gave him the epinephrine. Then, Dr. Feinstein said the most frightening thing I've heard from any of the doctors we've seen. He said that Dr. Boyer thinks Dylan should have a cardiac evaluation.

Needless to say, I panicked. Now, they think something is wrong with Dylan's heart?! Dr. Feinstein was very reassuring, though. He said he didn't think anything would come of it, but they just wanted him to be evaluated to be on the safe side and to see if there was a reason for the desaturation episode. I guess we'll be getting a referral to a cardiologist. He also has no idea why his breathing is still so bad – he thinks it's most likely an upper respiratory infection –, and his assessment said "I am hopeful this will improve over time." Yeah, you and me both. He did suggest that we get a saline nebulizer to break up some of the mucus, so we picked one up on the way home. I gave him his first treatment tonight, but I guess it's too soon to tell if it will help.

As luck would have it, when we got home, I'd received an e-mail from Samantha. She was very helpful and gave me a list of several possible diagnoses that seemed to fit what I told her about Dylan's situation:

- Transposition of the great vessels
- Tracheal/esophageal fistula
- Vascular ring/sling

Now, I'm off to do some research and learn more about all of them. God helps those who help themselves, right?

Monday, April 17, 2006

We spent a few hours in the ER today. Dylan's symptoms – the breathing, choking, spitting up, trouble feeding – haven't subsided at all. Dr. Feinstein (ENT) suggested that we go to the children's emergency room and get him checked out. They took a chest x-ray, which was negative. They called in Dr. Karas, a pediatric ear, nose, and throat doctor, who did a nasopharyngeal scope and observed him for a while. Eventually, they decided that the breathing difficulty was due to an inflamed epiglottis, probably because of the laryngomalacia. They gave him a dose of steroids and told us to see Dr. Boyer (GI) because they thought increased reflux was at the bottom of the whole thing.

This is why I'm so frustrated. The ER doctor thinks he's having increased reflux, but the endoscopy he had previously showed no signs of reflux at all. Which is it? I feel like we just keep going around in circles, and no one has any answers for Dylan.

Meanwhile, my marriage is struggling for many reasons. I can only stretch myself so thin with an active two-year-old and Dylan with his multiple medical issues, which are the most pressing right now.

Friday, April 21, 2006

FINALLY, we're getting some relief. Dylan's symptoms have started to decrease, and things are going much better. He still has issues, but it's much better than before. Maybe the steroids he got at the ER have kicked in and made a difference. I really don't care what the reason is. I'm just so relieved that he's getting better.

On the down side, I called Dr. Boyer's (GI) office for an appointment and was given a date a month from now! I explained to the nurse that Dylan is still experiencing lots of problems. He is choking all the time, during and after I feed him, often causing his breathing to get worse. He also spits up and vomits constantly, but she said his breathing issues "weren't in their department", so they didn't need to see him again until the end of May. After all that we'd been through, you'd think Dr. Boyer would want to keep a closer eye on him. Apparently not. I felt like we were getting the brush-off, but there's not much I can do about that.

However, what I CAN do is get another opinion. I made an appointment with a pediatric gastroenterologist at a second children's medical center in Connecticut. All of my instincts tell me that something is seriously wrong with my son, and I'm determined to do whatever it takes to get him the help he needs. In the meantime, we see the cardiologist on Tuesday.

Saturday, April 22, 2006

Feeding Dylan is frustrating for both him and me. For one thing, he feeds so sporadically. One week, I can barely get him to take 8 oz. of formula a day; the next, he's up to 18 oz., and then goes right back down to next-to-nothing. How can I keep him hydrated when he just won't drink?

My grandmother had a suggestion. She said we should put baby pasta into his bottle to thicken the formula. Sounds about right for an Italian/Polish grandmother! She might have a point, though. I tried thickening his bottles with a little rice cereal, and it seems to be helping. The ratio of cereal to formula is pretty ridiculous. In fact, it's so thick that I've had to enlarge the openings in the nipples. I've got it down to a science now, but there really isn't anyone but me who can prepare his formula because it's gotten so damn complicated.

Even though I'm grateful that the thickened formula seems to be working, I keep coming back to the fact that THIS IS NOT NORMAL! A 4-month-old baby should not be on an adult dose of Prevacid, and I shouldn't have to work so hard to figure out meals that he won't choke on. I don't understand what's going on, but there's got to be an answer.

Tuesday, April 25, 2006

Today's entrant on the Parade of Doctors is Dr. Guitano, a pediatric cardiologist, who is to evaluate the desaturation incident that took place when Dylan had the endoscopy. I can't believe that was only two weeks ago! It seems like a lifetime has passed since then.

The good news is that, as the other doctors predicted, he found nothing wrong with Dylan's heart. We talked about his entire history and the various doctors he's seen (I've almost lost count!), and he examined Dylan and ran some tests, including an EKG and a cardiac ultrasound, otherwise known as an ECHO. Dr. Guitano said both tests showed that his heart is structurally normal. He discharged him completely, saying he had "no restrictions from a cardiovascular standpoint." Thank God! At least there's one thing we don't have to worry about.

Wednesday, April 26, 2006

Today we saw Dr. Hallisey, a pediatric gastroenterologist, for a second opinion. Here's something scary. Dylan has been taking 30 mg of Prevacid, which Dr. Hallisey said is toxic for a baby. Good to know! He decreased the dose to 15 mg, so let's hope there's been no damage from that.

He also said that vomiting twenty times a day is not normal, especially with all his other symptoms. NO KIDDING! He ordered a barium swallow for tomorrow, so maybe we'll get some answers from that.

After all the doctors we've seen, it was sadly comforting to have someone tell me that what we're going through is definitely not normal. It's obvious to me, but most of the doctors we've seen seem to take it pretty casually. I guess they wouldn't be so cavalier about it if Dylan was their child, and they were going through this with him.

Thursday, April 27, 2006

Now, I really don't know what to think. We went for the barium swallow. As the radiologist was looking at the screen, he asked me if I'd ever heard the term "vascular ring." I was somewhat familiar with it because it was one of the things Samantha mentioned, and I'd done a little research on it. It certainly hasn't been mentioned by any of the other doctors we've seen, but this radiologist seemed pretty sure that it's what we're dealing with. He said it means that Dylan's aorta is formed abnormally and that it somehow forms a circle around his esophagus, which can cause problems with breathing and swallowing. Completely scary, but it kind of makes sense and could explain everything. But, why didn't the cardiologist see that on the ECHO?

Anyway, Dr. Hallisey's report says the GI series showed that everything is normal from the standpoint of Dylan's stomach and bowels; but, he recommends a CT scan to find out about the vascular ring, so I guess we're back to the cardiologist to see what he thinks. I sent him a copy of the report.

As if my life wasn't stressful enough, I got pulled over by a police officer on the way to Hartford. I was running late, which is always the case these days. I was flying up Route 9 to get to the appointment on time. Mom kept telling me to slow down. All of a sudden - WHAM! There were the flashing lights. The officer came up to the car and started on the usual questions, but the scene was like something from a movie. Dylan hates the car, so he was screaming his lungs out. Mom was saying, "I told her to slow down." I guess I looked pretty beaten down because the guy completely let me off the hook! He told me to slow down and stay safe, and then we were back on our way. For once, my chaotic existence paid off!

Monday, May 1, 2006

Dr. Guitano (cardiologist) called me today. He brushed the whole vascular ring thing off. He said he thought the radiologist's report "wasn't completely accurate" and told me not to worry about it. Seriously? A doctor tells me that my son might have a heart abnormality, and I'm not supposed to worry about that? I explained that Dylan's respiratory distress was increasing, but he still didn't think there was a problem and saw no need to see Dylan again.

So . . . I don't know what to think. The idea of a heart defect is incredibly scary. I did some research on the internet tonight, and it sounds EXACTLY like Dylan. The list of symptoms is like reading his medical chart: difficulty with feeding, respiratory distress, stridor, high-pitched cough, choking, reflux, vomiting. The more I read, the more convinced I became that we'd finally hit on the problem; but the cardiologist should know best, right??

I don't want to become one of those people who think a Google search is as good as a medical degree, and I've never questioned the opinions of my doctors this much before. Dr. Guitano is very qualified and comes highly recommended, and he says Dylan's echocardiogram was normal and that he doesn't have a vascular ring. On the other hand, the radiologist is also a qualified professional; and he seemed pretty convinced that he might have a vascular ring. In the end, I have to trust my instincts as a mother, along with the fact that I SAW IT FOR MYSELF ON THE SCREEN!

I'm not letting this go. All my instincts tell me that we're onto something. After we got home, I called Samantha and asked if she could set me up with someone at her hospital in PA, and I'm also trying to get in with someone at Boston Children's.

Tuesday, May 2, 2006

More frustration! Samantha set me up with a contact at her hospital and gave my info to Natalie, the cardiac surgical nurse practitioner there. I spoke to her on the phone about scheduling a consult, but she said that without a referral from a pediatrician they wouldn't be able to see us until the middle of June. I got the same story from Boston Children's. This problem should be easily solved. I'll just get a referral from Dr. Barclay (pediatrician).

Monday, May 8, 2006

Dylan is continuing to get worse. We left a message for Dr. Barclay, asking her to facilitate an appointment in PA or at Boston Children's. I feel so helpless.

Thursday, May 11, 2006

Well, it's been four days; and we have not heard from Dr. Barclay (pediatrician) or anyone else about a referral or an appointment.

Today, I stopped by the office of a good friend and former boss, Dr. Dixon. My grand entrance into his office was preceded by a 4-foot projectile vomit from Dylan, barely missing the glass door I needed to walk through. Oh my, this is ridiculous! Dr. Dixon sees my distress and fatigue and offers to make a phone call to the children's hospital that we previously visited in New Haven to see if he can get Dylan in for a work-up immediately. The doctor he spoke to said we would be receiving a call later this afternoon to set everything up. Hope this works.

Today is our anniversary, so Matt and I went out for dinner. Even though things are stressful at home, I'd take any excuse for a night out. While we were eating, I got a call from Dr. Barclay. If I thought I was going to get any help from her, I couldn't have been more wrong. She said she'd spoken to Dr. Guitano (cardiologist), and they agreed that Dylan DOESN'T have a vascular ring. She said the radiologist was only suggesting that there might be something there, but it was unlikely. I tried to push her on it – after all, I saw that screen with my own eyes – but she got really stern with me and insisted that Dylan has nothing more than a severe case of reflux. She said I'd better learn how to deal with it, or I was going to ruin my life. I can't remember the last time I was that angry. I hung up on her and downed my whole glass of wine!

I can't believe that both she and Dr. Guitano are completely brushing off even the possibility of a heart issue. I mean, that radiologist is board-certified with tons of experience at an excellent children's hospital. But, instead of even considering the possibility, she just insists that all of these issues will go away with time.

I wish I could believe her, but my gut says that's not the case.

Friday, May 12, 2006

Another day of waiting. We still hadn't heard from the hospital and, of course, it's a Friday afternoon to boot! (We all know what happens on a Friday afternoon in any office.) I spoke with Dr. Dixon again, who suggested contacting his father, a pediatrician in Cleveland, to see what suggestion he might have to help us. Within a couple of hours, his dad called me with a referral to a cardiologist in Cleveland, so I called and left a message for that doctor.

The doctor called me back. Whoa, same day too! I described Dylan's symptoms and told him about the report from the barium swallow. In a ten-minute conversation, without even seeing Dylan, he said it sounded like a vascular ring and urged me to have Dylan evaluated immediately. I asked whether he'd be willing to see Dylan, and he said yes. It looks like we're going to Cleveland.

I hate going all the way to Ohio when we (supposedly) have perfectly capable doctors in Connecticut, but I've lost faith. We've been at this for more than five months now, and we're no closer to an answer for the little guy. He's suffering every day, and it's making our family life a nightmare. If it takes going to Cleveland – or San Francisco or Rome or Istanbul – that's what we're going to do!

It looks like Dylan and I will be going alone, at least at first. Matt wants to wait until he sees the schedule before he makes plans, so I guess Sydney will stay home with him and then stay with Mom when he joins us. I hate being away from Syd, especially since I'm not sure how long we'll be in Cleveland; but this seems like the best solution for everyone.

We leave tomorrow and Dylan will be admitted to the children's hospital in Cleveland on Sunday.

Sunday, May 14, 2006

Whew! I'm beat, but we're in Cleveland and settled into our room.

We got to the hospital this afternoon after an uneventful flight. For many reasons, I'm soooo glad we were able to take a private plane. The best thing was the very kind and helpful pilot. I had no idea what to expect, so I brought everything – toys for Dylan, pillows, even the giant memory foam wedge he's been sleeping on. That thing has been a God-send, since he chokes if he lies flat after he eats. If the routine here goes like it does at home, he'll be okay napping in a crib. But, since he always throws up and chokes at bedtime, I thought I'd be safe and bring the wedge.

That pilot was amazing! He took Dylan and me from the airport to the hospital and stayed with us until Dylan had been admitted, and we were safely settled into a room. It was probably a pretty amusing scene – me standing there in the admissions area looking like a pack mule with a suitcase, a car seat, Lamby, a bunch of toys, a couple of pillows, the big foam wedge, a baby, and an airline pilot. I doubt if the hospital staff sees that every day.

Monday, May 15, 2006

The radiologist was right! Dylan had another echocardiogram at the hospital today, and it showed *two* aortas that were almost equal in size! It was so clear that even I could see it. My baby will have surgery on Wednesday. Scary – but I have a good feeling about it.

I can tell that I'm not going to get much rest while we're here. Dylan's room is really small, and it's right next to the nurses' station. There is a ton of activity all the time. The lights in the hallway are always on, and there are always people talking. Cardiac monitors are beeping 24 hours a day – just a lot of contained chaos. The room looks even smaller because I've got the giant foam wedge stuffed into Dylan's crib to make him more comfortable, and it gets even more cramped when I open the pull-out chair that will be my bed for the next few days. At least I can close the blinds on the window that looks out into the hallway to get a little privacy.

Dylan is adjusting pretty well to the new surroundings. Right now he's lying on his back in the crib with his Lamby over his eyes, sleeping soundly. Glad someone can.

Dylan has already made friends with all the staff, and he's only thrown up on two nurses so far! However, he's successfully blasted almost every square inch of the floor of our new "home." Good thing he's cute.

Tuesday, May 16, 2006

Lots of waiting today during all the pre-op testing. We took several stroller rides and watched a lot of Baby Einstein videos. This hospital has a great Child Life Department that offers everything imaginable for patients and their families. We borrowed a swing from there, which Dylan really likes.

My meals today were less than desirable, though – cafeteria food for breakfast, a granola bar for lunch, and mac and cheese from the vending machine for dinner. Yum! At least the coffee is good. It seems to be the mainstay at every meal.

All the waiting has given me a lot of time to think, and the thing that keeps coming back to me is my anger at Dr. Barclay (pediatrician). I'm frustrated with a lot of the doctors we've seen because no one seemed to take Dylan's problems seriously, but she's at the top of my list. She's his primary care doctor and has been following his case since January. I decided that rather than just sitting here seething about it maybe I'd feel better if I took some action, so I wrote her a letter telling her that Dylan would no longer be her patient. I tried to hold my temper and be professional, but I did make it clear that a mere four days after our last conversation – the night she called while Matt and I were at dinner and was so dismissive – Dylan was in the hospital awaiting surgery for the VERY CONDITION SHE WAS SURE HE DIDN'T HAVE.

I could have put it in the mailbox, but I sent it overnight by UPS. Just because.

Wednesday, May 17, 2006

Surgery day is finally over. Dylan was a little champ this morning while we were waiting for them to come for him. About 11:00 a.m., it was almost time for him to go. I was playing with him in my lap when I looked up and saw Matt standing in the doorway. How nice of him to join us.

Anyway, the procedure appears to have been a success. Dr. Henzin (cardiothoracic surgeon) said Dylan had a type of vascular ring called a double aortic arch, and he was able to fix it with no complications. Thank God!

Maggie, the cardiothoracic surgical nurse practitioner, said we need to follow up with a pulmonologist because Dylan's trachea didn't "pop out" like it should have, and it has probably sustained some damage from all this; but he's on the road to recovery. Several times she emphasized that we should follow up and get another bronchos-copy . . . but, right now, I need to sleep!

Thursday, May 18, 2006

I got to the ICU really early this morning to see Dylan. When I walked in, I could barely make out the shape of my baby. OMG! I've never seen so much equipment! There were monitors above the crib, tubes coming from the wall, and a suction machine hanging from his bed with tubes filled with blood coming from his little body. He had lines in both of his arms, two in his neck, a mask on his face; and he was in RESTRAINTS! I was terrified. Lamby, though, was right beside him.

Gradually, various staff members cycled through and pieced the story together for me. It seems that my little guy gave them an experience they won't soon forget. Apparently, he became very aggressive during the night. And, as he woke up, in between doses of his pain meds, he objected to all the things that were invading his body. He pulled out the central line from his neck and an IV from his arm, and he was even tugging at his chest tube. This child is five months old!

On a positive note, sometime during the night, he learned to roll from his back onto his tummy. That's a pretty good milestone, especially just six hours after surgery; so, good for him.

As the day went on, another concern came up. Dylan's systolic blood pressure is over 200. They've been giving him meds to get it down, but nothing is working so far. The cardiologist wants to wait it out for now. If there is no improvement by tomorrow, he'll want to do more tests.

Saturday, May 20, 2006

We were supposed to get discharged today, but that didn't happen. Yesterday, Dylan started to vomit again. Because I'm so used to that, I wasn't too concerned. Then, all of a sudden, I was the one who needed to vomit! THAT I'm not used to.

I was so sick. I begged to go back to the hotel room, so Matt stayed with Dylan. I spent the next twelve hours on the bathroom floor. I don't remember ever being that miserable.

This morning I dragged myself out of bed, feeling not great but okay, and headed to the hospital. When I got to the room, Matt was curled up in a ball on the couch. . HE has it now! What a mess. And, there was Dylan – hanging out in his crib, watching a movie.

Anyway, his discharge was postponed because he has to keep food down for twenty-four hours before they'll let him go; so we're here for at least another night.

Monday, May 22, 2006

Dylan is getting discharged, and we're going home!!!! It looks like we'll finally have a normal family life with two healthy, happy children.

Thursday, May 25, 2006

I've been thinking about which pediatric practice we should use, since we've cut ties with Dr. Barclay. I've decided to go back to our first one. Even though Dylan is better since the surgery, we've been assured that there are a ton of things that can still go wrong, most of them related to something called tracheomalacia and tracheal stenosis, which apparently could cause him to need a surgical reconstruction of his trachea. That would mean he'd have to be intubated for at least a week! Can you imagine? The poor little guy has been through so much already, so it breaks my heart that he might have to endure even more, simply because a bunch of doctors were too quick to dismiss his symptoms and my concerns. Since his most recent bronchoscopy indicated that he does indeed have tracheal abnormalities, he might very well have to have surgery sooner rather than later. It's clear that he still has respiratory issues. Given his luck so far in his short life, I'd be shocked if he DIDN'T need more surgery. Everything else has gone wrong, so why shouldn't that?

As grateful as I am that he's doing better since the surgery, I'm still angry and frustrated that the many doctors we've seen – starting with Dr. Barclay (pediatrician) – didn't look past a "fussy" infant and a "paranoid" mother and diagnose him earlier. He always looked well and didn't have "failure to thrive", so they all thought he was fine. According to everything I've read – which is a lot since I've become a bit obsessed by all of this – he should have had surgery by the time he was three months old. Early intervention has been absolutely proven to lessen the damage caused by his condition, so now we just have to hope that the residual effects of all this will be minimal.

To be honest, I'm also a little disappointed in myself. I KNEW something was wrong with him. Although I'm glad I was persistent – and

I'm especially glad I pursued the doctor in Cleveland – looking back, I wish I'd pushed even harder. The thing is it's hard to fight the health care system. They stick together and can be pretty intimidating, not perhaps intentionally; but there's no question that it's hard to argue with them.

On the other hand, they might have all that education and knowledge and high-tech equipment, but I've got something they don't have – a mother's natural intuition and instincts. I know my child. I observe him 24/7. I know what's normal and what isn't. And, I feel guilty because I let Dylan down by not pushing even harder than I did. Matt thought I was pushing too hard anyway; but now I know it wasn't enough, so I feel guilty. I also feel sad that Dylan had to suffer – and might have to suffer more in the future – because a dozen doctors failed him.

So, I think we'll go back to the original pediatric practice where the hours are longer, the location is closer, and there is more than one doctor available when you need help. I hope it's the right decision, because I really need to find a doctor who gives a crap.

Wednesday, May 31, 2006

Got a handwritten note from Dr. Barclay (pediatrician) today expressing her "regret that I was unable to meet your needs at this time". That's an understatement! Weird thing is that I also got a call from an assistant to the physician Dr. Dixon spoke with back on May 8th. She was calling to set up Dylan's MRI. I could only utter the words, "We are all set. Thanks, though." STUNNED!

Tuesday, June 6, 2006

Here's something disturbing. I've been trying to collect all the records on Dylan's medical history over the past six months. I contacted Dr. Guitano's (cardiologist) office to ask for a copy of his evaluation note, the echocardiogram report, and a copy of the actual echocardiogram.

Well, today I got a call from his office telling me that I can't get the actual echocardiogram because they don't have it anymore. It seems that they "reused" the tape. They erased Dylan's results and taped over it with someone else's test. How is that possible? We're talking about one of the country's major hospitals! This can't possibly be standard procedure there. It's not like the test took place years and years ago. It was just a few weeks ago! I have to say that I find it an incredible coincidence that Dr. Guitano clearly screwed up Dylan's diagnosis, and the evidence has suddenly disappeared!

I still have the note he dictated from his appointment with Dylan back in April – the one in which he said there was nothing wrong with his heart. But, it would be nice to see the actual echocardiogram to see if it really shows nothing wrong (which is unlikely, since the other doctors – who aren't even cardiologists! – saw the problem) or if he missed something incredibly obvious.

Monday, June 12, 2006

Oh, how irony works…I received a Patient Satisfaction Survey to fill out in regard to my appointment with Dr. Guitano (cardiologist). Here's my chance!

Monday, June 19, 2006

Dylan is starting to sound junky again, and he seems to be having a bit of difficulty breathing. I called the pediatrician's office because the surgical team in Cleveland made it very clear that we need to jump on anything like this immediately. Dylan fails so fast that it's critical to begin treatment the minute things start to go south.

They saw us really quickly but didn't do anything. The doctor said he's fine and just has a small cold. No treatment, no suggestions, no nothing. Hello? Has anyone even read his (very extensive) chart? Even in my sleep, I can tell when he's going to crash because we've been through this more than a few times already.

I'll give it one more day. If there's no improvement, I'll pull out the guns.

Tuesday, June 20, 2006

And, here I am again at the pediatrician's office! Now Dylan has a fever, and he looks horrible. Coughing constantly and mild respiratory distress . . . same old story.

During the initial intake with the nurse, I went through his whole history, including the surgery he had just a month ago. I couldn't believe I had to go through it AGAIN, like it's not in his damn chart. Well, no sooner than I sat down, the Head Honcho came in and took over. Now THAT is service. He told me that he will be handling Dylan's case personally from now on, so I'm feeling a little more reassured.

I'm really struggling over the idea of pursuing a lawsuit over all of this. I'm not a litigious person by nature, but we've been through so much with Dylan; and it's clear that mistakes were made, especially by Dr. Guitano (cardiologist). I just feel like someone needs to address it.

In response to the Patient Satisfaction Survey form, I wrote a letter to the president of the medical group to tell him what happened with the so-called normal echocardiogram and its subsequent erasing. I doubt anything will come of it. Those guys seem to stick up for each other, no matter what; but I had to say something. Dylan doesn't have anybody else to stick up for him.

Friday, June 23, 2006

I received a call today from the president of the medical group. WOW! Was I surprised! (I guess he read my letter.) After briefly listening to my complaints, he abruptly reassured me that he would look into this and get back to me. I must have struck a nerve to get a response so quickly. Or, does he really read his mail every day?

Monday, June 26, 2006

I received a call today from some woman who works with the medical group's president. I was informed that Dr. Guitano (cardiologist) no longer works at the hospital or with the cardiology group. (Is this karma or a coincidence?) He now works for an insurance company. Oddly enough, it is MY insurance company! Don't think I didn't call them immediately and let them know about all the mistakes that have been made since Dylan's birth and all of their money that has been wasted. Obviously, it didn't do any good; but I felt better for having gotten that off my chest.

Sunday, June 25, 2006

I'm so frustrated.

Despite everything we've been through, including the surgery, Dylan STILL isn't feeding properly. Before the surgery, he was vomiting up to 30 times a day. Now, he's not vomiting as much; but he just doesn't want to eat. What could be wrong now???

Maybe we'll get some answers on Thursday. We're going in for a "feeding assessment" that will hopefully help us get to the bottom of this newest issue.

Thursday, June 29, 2006

Dylan had his feeding assessment today. First, they went over his entire medical history, including the vascular ring repair last month and the fact that the GI study didn't show any gastrointestinal issues that would explain the feeding problems. It's a good thing I keep such extensive records, because they wanted to know every detail of his feeding history – the names of his various formulas, when solid foods were introduced and what kind, amounts of everything he ate, and even the kind of bottle we used.

After going over all of that, they started working directly with him; and it was pretty interesting to watch. They put him in a high chair and tried feeding him some pureed bananas and Alimentum formula. Then, they just observed and recorded all his actions and reactions. They noted that he really wanted to eat and got upset when they withheld food and that all his reflexes, coordination, and so on were normal.

Their conclusion is that all the vomiting before his surgery has caused Dylan's oral and taste sensations to be out of whack. That seems to make sense. The solution they presented is that we learn to feed him differently, and they had quite a few suggestions. For example, when I offer him a spoonful of food, I'm supposed to use my finger to support his chin and direct the spoon toward the sides of his mouth, rather than the center. When I offer the spoon toward the center of his mouth, I'm supposed to gently push it down on his tongue. All of this will require some practice for me and a learning curve for Dylan, too; but it all seems reasonable and do-able.

They also think he's ready to start using a cup. In a couple of months, we can try him on meats. We're still avoiding soy because of a possible allergy, and I'm supposed to introduce new foods gradually, so we can be on the lookout for other allergies.

I feel like we made some progress today. Now, it's just a matter of practicing the new feeding techniques until we go back for a follow-up visit in September.

Wednesday, July 19, 2006

We had a follow-up bronchoscopy yesterday, with Dr. Bennett, the new pulmonologist. There was absolutely no improvement since the surgery, which is quite concerning. Eighty per cent of his airway is closed off in two areas. Oh, boy. This was not what I wanted to hear. We're going back next week to meet with the pulmonary therapist to establish what they call a "sick plan" for when he starts having problems. Wonder how much that will entail.

At least I do not have to search for doctors anymore, since we got established with a cardiologist and a pulmonologist for follow-up care before we left the hospital in Cleveland. Soon we'll have seen every pediatric specialist in Connecticut!

Saturday, July 22, 2006

I decided to write letters to my "favorite" docs. Maybe they will better understand what we have gone through over the past few months. Well, maybe more just to clear my head.

LETTER 1:

Dear Dr. . ███████,

Approximately six months ago, I transferred Dylan's care to you. He was six weeks old at that time; and it was obvious to me that Dylan had a medical problem, which was not being addressed.

It is extremely frustrating, and even sad, to review your notes and to remember my everyday worries as his symptoms played out. We all know hind-sight makes many issues clearer; however, here is a newborn child who is presenting with choking and coughing and feeding problems that continue to pose problems on a daily basis; and, yet, you failed to look past the diagnosis of "reflux". At a particularly difficult time, when I independently sought outside help in the ███ Pediatric Emergency Room on 2/14/06, your presence trumped my goal and interrupted an independent evaluation. Furthermore, your E.R. note from that day said "I'm not sure why she came to the E.R. Apparently, the baby was extremely fussy today".

While you were attempting to expedite an appointment with Dr. ███████ for a G.I. consult, even into March and April, your progress notes for Dylan refer to "choking on bottles"; "noisy chest", "looks uncomfortable", "increased WOB", "increased throwing up", and most notably, "insp/exp stridor". Did you not even once suspect that something other than reflux might be going on with all these symptoms? Or, did you write me off as just another "neurotic mother" because of all the calls? It always came down to reflux and formula and deferring to that elusive G.I. consult.

As you now know, with a simple barium swallow study, Dylan was diagnosed with a vascular ring. On 5/17/06, at age five months, he had division of ligamentum arteriosus and division of left aortic arch. His pre-operative/post-operative diagnosis was double aortic arch causing esophageal and tracheal stenosis.

You may or may not know that there are post-operative symptoms that can take months or years to resolve. Many of the postoperative symptoms are related to the presence of tracheomalacia. Some infants must undergo tracheal reconstruction with placement of an endotracheal tube for at least one week! Dylan's follow-up bronchoscopy indicates that he does, indeed, have tracheomalacia with involvement of the right main stem bronchus. He could be a surgical candidate in the immediate future. Without surgery, his respiratory status is guarded.

The medical literature says, "In infants who present with feeding disorders, spitting, or dyspnea, congenital vascular anomalies should be high on the differential diagnosis list". We are extremely fortunate that Dylan's problem was identified, albeit after months of pushing "the system", and that his surgery went well. This could have had a different outcome. And, although we are still facing another major surgical procedure, we are hopeful that he will have minimal residual pulmonary symptoms as he grows. Obviously, the sooner the diagnosis is made the less damage there is. Dylan should have had surgery by age three months.

Yes, I'm a bit angry, frustrated, and disappointed that I didn't push even more than I did. I remember trying to accept the explanations while always feeling in my heart that there was more to this picture. This is the guilt and sadness that I live with each day, feeling now that I let my child down by not taking the situation into my own hands as I wanted to. You try to respect the professionals and work with them, but sometimes a mother's gut feeling and 24-7 observations are worth more than a medical degree; and, when a child presents with what-seems-to-be-routine symptoms, the answer can't always be "reflux" or "viral infection" or "he'll-grow-out-of-it" explanations.

I am very grateful for Dylan's chance at a normal life, recognizing that other children endure lifetime physical and mental illnesses. I can only hope that this can be a learning experience for those of you who missed the opportunity to diagnose a cardiac anomaly in a newborn.

Sincerely,

████████████

LETTER 2:

Dear Dr. ████ :

Dylan was initially seen by you in your office on 3/08/06 for, according to your note, "irritability, vomiting and diarrhea". Your initial note also states "mother refers to constant irritability with choking spells soon after feeds".

In your Review of Systems (ROS) you noted: ENT: "stridor" and GI: "vomiting, choking spells, irritability". Your assessment was 1) GERD, 2) Milk protein sensitivity, and 3) Laryngomalacia. Your plan was to 1) Increase Prevacid to15 mg. b.i.d.; may use antacids for irritability, 2) Extensive re-assurance provided to the mother, 3) Follow-up in 3 months.

I called your office on 3120106 reporting an episode of "black flecks in spit up" and "yellow, seedy stools". By phone, you prescribed Gaviscon. On 3/30/06, now with a report of three episodes of coffee-ground emesis, you left a phone message for me to add Carafate and to continue Prevacid. There was no mention of a follow-up appointment sooner than the "three months" set on 3/8/06.

On 4/03/06, Dylan was seen by Dr. ███████ who made note of "increased vomiting", another "episode of coffee-ground emesis", "decreased intake", "not great diapers" (obviously, relative to intake) "looks uncomfortable", "chest noisy". There was a call to you on 4/03/06 and 4/05/06 and 4/06/06. You and Dr. ███████ were supposed to be talking to each other. Your answer to the phone note on 4/06/06 was "plan endoscopy".

On 4/10/06, you performed an upper endoscopy on Dylan. Your postoperative conversation with me stated that everything looked good. No evidence of ulcer or bleeding. No signs of reflux on scoping. You did mention that he had a "pretty good S-curve in the esophagus" and that "it's probably a hiatus hernia, which will stretch out as he grows". Routine follow-up was to be at age 6 months.

In the Recovery Room, following endoscopy, a nurse reported a "little episode occurred in the O.R. requiring a vaso-nebulizer treatment" and that "Dylan would have to remain in Recovery for an extra hour" because of this. I'm surprised that you failed to mention this "little episode" to me, considering that I learned it was a de-saturation issue during intubation.

Dylan's respiratory distress increased following endoscopy. Dr. ▮▮▮▮▮ and Dr. ▮▮▮ met us in the ▮▮ Emergency Room on 4/17/06. It was discussed then what Dr. ▮▮▮▮▮ had learned about a recommendation for a cardiology appointment relating to the events of the OR. Why had it not been scheduled yet? (Imagine my surprise at that question?) Apparently, you had a conversation with him and mentioned how the oxygen saturation dropped during intubation and that Dylan should have a cardiology consult. You never relayed this information to me or Dr. ▮▮▮▮. You also failed to note your findings on endoscopy; i.e. "S-curve"; suspect "hiatus hernia", and the fact that the patient had an episode of de-saturation during intubation. O.R. notes are usually very precise and thorough.

On 4/18/06, a phone message to you from me reported "reflux" was worse. You attributed it to intubation/procedure. By 4/20/06, with no change in his G.I. and respiratory symptoms, I transferred to G.I. at ▮▮▮▮▮▮▮▮▮▮▮▮▮▮▮▮▮▮▮▮. A next-day barium swallow gave us the answer.

Dylan was born with a vascular ring. On 5/17/06, at age 5 months, he had division of ligamentum arteriosus and division of the left aortic arch at ▮▮▮▮▮▮▮▮▮▮▮▮▮▮▮▮▮▮▮▮▮ ▮▮▮▮▮▮▮. His pre- and post-operative diagnosis was double aortic arch causing esophageal and tracheal stenosis. The medical literature says, "In infants who present with feeding disorders, spitting, or dyspnea, congenital vascular anomalies should be high on the differential diagnosis list".

This anomaly isn't common for sure. However, in retrospect, had a little more effort been put into sifting through his symptoms and/or picking up on some pretty unusual findings, like an "S-curve" on endoscopy, Dylan might have been diagnosed earlier on. The delay in diagnosis has left him with tracheomalacia, leaving him wide-open for pulmonary problems in the future unless surgically corrected.

A mother's observation of her child should be respected. Reflux cannot always be the answer for G.I. symptoms in babies. Hopefully, you will look "outside the box" when another mother reaches out to you for help. We all know that Dylan's outcome could have been much different if I didn't continue to push through the system for an answer.

Sincerely,

█████████

Friday, September 8, 2006

Sydney started pre-K this week . . . and Dylan has a cold. Of course, this being Dylan, it's not just any cold. He sounds like he's under water when he breathes. The pediatrician wants us to bypass their office for anything respiratory and go directly to the pulmonologist, so I made the call. They started him on nebulizer treatments of Albuterol and Atrovent, along with chest percussion four times a day. Now, I just have to figure out how to get a 9-month-old boy to sit still for six treatments a day. . .and build on a new room to house the pharmacy I seem to have in my house now.

Monday, October 2, 2006

Just got home from a CT scan with Dylan. We've got a surgical consult at Mass General tomorrow, and we need to bring this with us, in addition to the bronchoscopy results.

This experience wasn't fun for anyone. Because he's only 10 months old, they had to sedate him so he wouldn't move in the CT scanner. They gave him some sort of sleeping concoction, but it didn't do the trick; and he was still too wide awake to put him into the machine. After 30 minutes, they started talking about rescheduling because they had a lot of tests scheduled for today; but I put my foot down. No way am I coming back and, besides, I need this for our appointment tomorrow; and I'm NOT rescheduling that.

So . . . I grabbed a radiation blanket and covered up, picked up Dylan (who was by no means awake like normal), and put him on the table. Then, I climbed onto the table on my hands and knees (in a short skirt – not the best wardrobe choice for this kind of activity) and held him still. The girls raised their eyebrows and said, "You sure?" Oh yeah, I'm sure.

Looking back, we must have made quite the spectacle. I'm sure my shenanigans made their day and gave them something to talk about for weeks to come – the crazy mom who climbed into the CT scanner with her baby. But it was worth a little humiliation because I got home with my CT in hand!

Tuesday, October 3, 2006

We had our appointment at Mass General today with a pediatric surgeon, Dr. Bosco. He went over Dylan's entire history with me. After much ado, he concluded that there is nothing to be done right now. He looked at the chest CT we had done yesterday and said there was no sign of pneumonia or anything else, other than the tracheomalacia. He said that nothing was impinging on his esophagus to explain the continuing cough and other issues. He doesn't think his continuing symptoms warrant another bronchoscopy, or even x-rays at the moment; so I guess we'll keep soldiering on.

Wednesday, October 11, 2006

I decided I can't just sit around and do nothing, so I called Samantha about getting a consult with someone in PA – at her hospital. I want to talk to someone about the recommendations we got from the Cleveland surgical team, as well as Dylan's latest bronchoscopy results. She thought it was a good idea, so she's putting me in touch with a cardiothoracic surgeon to see if Dylan needs to be followed for a possible tracheal reconstruction.

Friday, October 13, 2006

Got an appointment set up with the surgeon in PA. We'll fly down there in two weeks. Lots of waiting and wondering...

Friday, October 27, 2006

It's been hours since we left Pennsylvania, but my blood is still boiling.

Today was our appointment with the "amazing" surgeon. We flew down there in the morning, got to the hospital, and sat in the waiting room for an hour. Finally, we got called back; and 15 minutes later we were out the door again.

I couldn't believe it. This guy took a quick glance at Dylan and said, "He looks fine. Why are you here?"

I gave him Dylan's records, but he never even looked at them. He asked a couple of questions and sent us on our way. No help, no suggestions, and absolutely no compassion. He acted like we were wasting his valuable time, and he couldn't have cared less about Dylan.

I'm so discouraged. Things are deteriorating between Matt and me, and I'm no closer to getting help for Dylan. I really don't know where to turn next.

Saturday, December 9, 2006

It's Dylan's first birthday. We had a bunch of close friends and family over to celebrate. It was nice to relax and help the little guy open presents. Dylan was so exhausted at the end – he grabbed Lamby and fell asleep before I could change him. Oh well, it is his birthday!

Saturday, December 16, 2006

Happy Holidays. . . at least to most people. My peaceful Christmas shopping trip with the kids turned sour when Dr. Barclay (former pediatrician) walked into the same store. I couldn't believe it. What are the odds?

She paused for a second when she saw me. Then, she came toward me, stopping as she realized how tense I was getting. I just don't have a good poker face. I thought she'd just move on, but she said, "Dylan looks great! Glad everything is fine."

FINE? I was dumbfounded. I said, "You have no idea what we go through on a daily basis, but I'm so happy to be his mother." I wanted to say more, but what good would it do? There's no way to make her understand.

The encounter was brief, but it brought back all those angry feelings from last spring. That was the end of my shopping trip. Seeing her killed my holiday mood, so we left the store and went home.

Friday, January 12, 2007

Well, I actually did it. The kids and I moved out today. I hate the fact that my marriage is ending, but I'm also looking forward to living in what I hope will be a more peaceful home.

The house is nice, and it will be great to live right next door to Dad. It will be a while before we're really settled; but, even though the kids are in bed, I'm too tired to do any more tonight. Hope to make a lot of progress over the weekend.

Saturday, January 13, 2007

Well, a miracle has occurred. I was worried that the kids would be upset about the move; but Dylan actually slept all the way through the night last night! First time EVER! I guess the stress of the past few months has been affecting all of us.

Wednesday, January 24, 2007

The nurse came over for Dylan's monthly RSV vaccination today. This is the third one, and I guess he'll have to have them through the spring or as long as he's at such a high risk of respiratory infections. I'm not sure how much good they're doing, since he's still sick all the time; but, who knows? Maybe he'd be even worse without them, especially with these New England winters.

Thursday, February 1, 2007

Dylan is back on oral steroids again. His symptoms have been increasing over the past couple of days, so I called the pulmonologist today. At least I don't have to take him into the office anymore, except for scheduled check-ups. I just call. They take care of the prescription over the phone, which is helpful, although, I'm a little surprised the doctor doesn't want to actually see him.

The steroids help, but I hate it when he has to take them because they make him CRAZY. He barely sleeps at all, he's unbelievably irritable, and he looks like he's been out binging all night. It makes it that much harder to do his nebulizer treatments, which is bad because we've got to increase them until his symptoms subside. Going to be a rough few days.

Wednesday, February 21, 2007

My mini-vacation is over, and I'm more exhausted that I was before we left.

Sydney, Dylan, my nanny Carrie, and I took advantage of the long holiday weekend to spend a few days with Dad in Florida. I was really looking forward to getting away and resting a bit, but it was not to be. Dylan's health started getting worse almost immediately. He stopped eating and drinking. By the third day, he had a fever of 103 and was wheezing like crazy, so off we went to the ER in Palm Beach. I expected to be there forever; but we were lucky to get the names of a couple of specialists, so we were only there for five hours. We left there with a diagnosis of double pneumonia, two large antibiotic shots in each leg, and yet more prescriptions.

He's better now, but I need another vacation.

Thursday, March 1, 2007

Dylan had his first speech therapy appointment today. Along with all his other issues, it's become noticeable that he's just not talking like he should at this age – a few words at best – so, hopefully, this will help. He seemed to like the therapist. That's a good start.

Thursday, April 5, 2007

Dylan's speech therapist thinks he might have some sensory percep-
tion issues, so she is giving us a referral to an occupational therapist.
He's only been working with the speech therapist for a month, but
we've already seen progress.

Tuesday, May 8, 2007

And the list of health care professionals grows yet again. Today we had our first consultation with a holistic nutritionist, who is going to work on clearing up Dylan's horrible eczema. The poor kid's eyes keep swelling shut. I'm worried that he'll have permanent scars on his trunk and legs and even his cute little face. Not only does it look awful, but it makes him miserable. It's just one more thing for the kid to put up with.

Thursday, September 6, 2007

Another scary night. I woke up about 1:00 a.m. to the sound of muted crying and choking, so I ran into Dylan's room. Whoa! He was coughing and literally gasping for air; and, of course, he was in a state of total panic.

I stayed as calm as I could and grabbed his Albuterol inhaler, thinking that would be the fastest remedy; but it didn't work. By that time, he was crying hysterically and bucking so hard I could barely hold onto him.

I set up the nebulizer and gave him a treatment, which helped more; and his breathing got a bit more normal, so he stopped crying, thank God. Poor kid was terrified, and so was his mom.

Even though he was better, he was still really uncomfortable; so I stayed on the floor holding him the rest of the night while he held lambies. Oh, yeah. There are two of them now - one for each hand. He was ripping the original one apart, so I bought another, thinking I'd give it to him if the first one came totally apart. Well, Sydney found it in a closet and gave it to him. Now, he won't let go of either one. It's pretty cute, and they do seem to bring him comfort.

I spent the rest of the night wondering what on earth was going on. Could he be developing asthma now? That's sure what it seemed like.

Needless to say, we were in the pediatrician's office first thing this morning. They gave him more breathing treatments and will see him again next week.

Monday, September 10, 2007

Dylan is FINALLY starting to bounce back from that weird asthma-like incident last week. The pediatrician sent him for x-rays on Friday, and he's had a ton of breathing treatments. No one is really sure what happened, though.

I just hope it was a one-time thing.

Monday, December 10, 2007

No Christmas tree for us, at least not in the house. I brought it in, got it into the stand, and we all worked together to decorate it. It really looked beautiful.

Then, within 48 hours, Dylan's eyes were swelled shut; and he couldn't stop scratching. It would appear that he's allergic to greenery. Why am I not surprised?

Clearly, it couldn't stay inside, so I moved it out to the deck – decorations and all. Hope the neighbors enjoy it!

Wednesday, April 2, 2008

I've never been so glad to see winter coming to an end. Dylan has been through hell and back since November. I've lost count of the number of sinus infections he's had. Just as one starts to get better, another one hits him. Add a few bouts of pneumonia on top of that, and you've got a recipe for pure misery.

And, the medications! Six consecutive weeks of antibiotics, four rounds of oral steroids, not to mention the breathing treatments and other crap he's always on. We found out he's allergic to penicillin (and tree nuts!), but other antibiotics don't seem to bother him, at least for now. Surely, it can't be good for him to be on so much medication, though.

He's scheduled to get tubes in his ears in a couple of days, so hopefully that – plus some warmer spring weather – will stop the constant infections.

Wednesday, April 16, 2008

The strangest and most wonderful thing has happened. All of a sudden, just out of the blue, Dylan's speech has improved dramatically; and he's started speaking in complete sentences!

This all happened right after he got the tubes in his ears a few days ago. Turns out he couldn't hear well at all; so, naturally, that impeded his speech development. Go figure!

Of course, now Sydney says he needs to shut up; but she's really happy her little brother can communicate better and be more of a playmate. As far as I'm concerned, he can talk all he wants. He's probably built up a lot of things he needs to say!

Saturday, April 19, 2008

When Dylan came home this afternoon, he was wheezing like crazy. I asked Matt for his inhaler. He went through his pockets but couldn't find it. "I guess I forgot to bring it," he said. Are you kidding me?

Looks like I need to keep duplicates of everything now.

Tuesday, May 6, 2008

Another weekend away from home and another medical issue. Dylan came home with pink eye in both eyes. It couldn't have been more obvious. No doctor visit. No medication. Hmmmm.

I'm so tired of feeling like I'm all alone in this.

Monday, June 2, 2008

It happened again! Dylan came home sick with a temp of 101.3. I was called for advice, but no Tylenol was given. Not sure why not. That was my instruction.

I don't know why I should be surprised anymore, but somehow I still am.

Saturday, August 9, 2008

Everything has been a whirlwind since Mike and I got married. We're slowly getting settled into a new house and getting more familiar with Stonington. Sydney misses her friends, but she'll be starting kindergarten in a couple of weeks and will make new ones then.

Let's hope this new start will be good for all of us.

Wednesday, September 17, 2008

Dylan has another respiratory infection. I called the pulmonologist, who called in another round of steroids but, of course, didn't want to see Dylan.

I think I'm going to look for a new lung specialist. I think this girl is competent, but it upsets me that I never get to talk to her when Dylan has a problem; and she NEVER wants to actually see him. At first, I thought it was convenient that I didn't have to haul off to the office every time the kid has a problem, but this has gone on for nearly a year now; and I just think it's a pretty inferior way to run a practice, especially when your patients are children. This is Dylan's fifth round of steroids in just a few months, so you'd think his doctor would want to actually examine him instead of just calling the pharmacy!

Friday, September 26, 2008

Got the name of a new pulmonologist today. Turns out the mother of one of Sydney's school friends knew someone, so I called for an appointment. They can't see us until November, but that's okay. It's not like his current doctor ever sees him anyway.

Thursday, October 9, 2008

Dylan had a check-up with the cardiologist in Hartford today, and I noticed something really cute and endearing. He and I have been to so many medical appointments that we've got a little routine down. We know exactly where to park, where the elevator is, what floor to go to, which way to turn when we get off the elevator . . . I think both of us could do it blindfolded. We're even on a first-name basis with the staff.

The weirdest thing, though, is that we've developed a special connection that's a result of everything we've been through since he was born. I guess it's my job as a mom to know what he needs; but, even though he's just a toddler, he seems to know what I need, too. He seems to sense how I'm feeling without me having to say a word. Whatever the future holds, I think he and I will always have a special bond; and I'm so grateful for that.

Sunday, November 2, 2008

I'm sitting here looking at my little Liam! It's hard to believe he's here already. He's just beautiful. The birth yesterday went so much more smoothly than Dylan's did. This family really feels complete now.

Thursday, November 13, 2008

Saw the new pulmonologist today. Dr. Palazzo spent TWO HOURS with us! Pretty amazing, after not even being able to get the last doc on the phone.

She was absolutely horrified when she learned how much medication Dylan has been taking, especially the steroids. I've thought for a while that all these meds must be wreaking havoc on his little body, so it was reassuring that she agreed. She said he's starting to exhibit signs of Cushing's Syndrome, which is a result of prolonged exposure to certain kinds of drugs. So, that is yet ANOTHER thing he has to contend with.

She cut his meds to the bare minimum and wants to have his tonsils and adenoids removed because she thinks they're restricting his air flow. She recommended we go back and see Dr. Karas, the pediatric ENT, who had put tubes in Dylan's ears last spring. Turns out he's also one of the doctors who saw Dylan when we took him to the ER back when he was just four months old! Dr. Palazzo said she'd do a bronchoscopy at the same time Dr. Karas takes out the tonsils. She thinks it's time we got another look at his trachea.

Honestly, how do medically ignorant families survive in the health care system? I'm a nurse, and it's hard enough for me to navigate the whole mess. I'm sure a lot of people just give up. There really has to be an easier way.

Sunday, November 16, 2008

Kids spent the weekend away from me; and, of course, it didn't end well for Dylan. Turns out he didn't have any of his breathing treatments, so he missed six Pulmicort and three DuoNeb treatments; and he didn't even get a hit of Albuterol before running around.

Monday, January 12, 2009

Early morning; long day. Dylan, both lambies, and I arrived in New Haven at 6:30 a.m. to have his tonsils and adenoids removed. Dr. Karas seems competent and caring. We've seen so many doctors in the past few years that they're all starting to blend together in my mind.

The surgery itself went well; but, of course, we got more bad news. Dr. Palazzo did a bronchoscopy that showed Dylan's airway 80% constricted in two places, and he has a lot of inflammation in his lungs. Can you imagine? It's amazing the poor little guy can breathe at all. Hopefully, today's procedure will help a little bit. They put him back on reflux meds, since the inflammation is a product of aspiration. How am I supposed to get these meds mixed and administered an hour before he eats when he wakes up starving at 6:00 a.m.? I'll figure it out.

This is still a fairly common surgery for kids and not especially complicated; but, with all Dylan has been through, I really hated having to do it. As usual, he was a trouper. He was groggy and thirsty and complaining about his throat being sore, but otherwise came through it fine.

We didn't get clearance to leave until nearly 7:00 p.m., and then it took another hour to get through the discharge process and all the paperwork. We were finally ready to head home at 8:00 p.m. Dylan was sound asleep with lambies by 9:15 p.m.; and, now, I'm off to bed, too.

Sunday, January 25, 2009

I want to scream. Or cry. Or both. Yeah, probably both.

Let's backtrack. Friday night, the kids were going away for the weekend. Dylan was sick (what's new, right?) so I was a little reluctant to let him go; but I was reassured that everything would be okay. So, I sent them off with care instructions and a list of phone numbers for all our doctors. Frankly, I was ready for a little break.

This afternoon, when I picked the kids up, I couldn't believe Dylan. He was so lethargic that he couldn't even get out of the car. I had to carry him. He clearly had a fever – his skin was on fire – and he was so dehydrated that his lips were cracked. I was so anxious to get him home that I didn't ask any questions. When I got back home, I checked him out immediately. His temp was 103.5, and his oxygen was down to 91%. The poor kid!

After I gave him some Tylenol, an Albuterol nebulizer treatment, some juice, and a lot of love and compassion; he went to sleep right away. I called to find out what had happened. I was told that Dylan hadn't eaten all weekend and barely drank anything, but he was "fine." Fine? Really?

I left a message at the pediatrician's office. Hopefully, we can get an early appointment tomorrow.

Monday, January 26, 2009

It's pneumonia. No surprise there. This happens every time he gets sick. We're back on antibiotics, pushing liquids, doing eight nebulizer treatments a day, and trying to avoid the hospital.

The poor guy is coughing so much it makes him vomit. I can't work or even give Sydney and Liam the attention they need because this home treatment plan consumes every minute of my time. Our only saving grace is The Backyardigans. Dylan watches an episode every time he has a breathing treatment, which gives me a little time to take care of the other kids and do a few things around the house. I definitely need to clone myself!

Sunday, March 1, 2009

Dylan is sick again; respiratory distress and a terrible cough, prob-ably not helped by the fact that once again he didn't have any of his medications. Two days without his meds and treatments is not a good thing for this kid. Unbelievable.

Saturday, March 7, 2009

Dylan is still sick: oxygen was 94%, and he had a 100 degree fever.

All these nebulizer treatments! I'm feeling they are not even working, but what's the alternative? I feel so badly for Dylan.

Sunday, May 3, 2009

And, once again, Dylan came home sicker than he was when he left here. He wasn't given his meds, even the antibiotics for his chest infection.

It's gotten to the point that I worry constantly. I can't enjoy my down time because I know I'll have to deal with the consequences later on but mostly hate to see Dylan feel so lousy.

Wednesday, July 15, 2009

I took Dylan for another bronchoscopy today, and we got yet more bad news. His airway is still 80 % constricted; and when they tested the inflammation in his lungs, the results were through the roof.

I can't say I was terribly surprised. The poor guy seems to be coughing and choking more recently, and his growth has slowed down noticeably.

We go back to Dr. Palazzo in a couple of weeks. She'll have today's results to consider, so we'll see whether she has any new ideas.

Tuesday, August 4, 2009

Dr. Palazzo is concerned about Dylan's airway and thinks it might be time to do a tracheal reconstruction. But, first she needs Dylan to get a CT scan and a G.I. workup. She's going to schedule the CT scan and has referred me to a Dr. Russell in Providence for a G.I. consult. Depending on the results, she'll probably send us to a thoracic surgeon to see what might be done to open up Dylan's airway. With an 80% constriction, I don't see how he breathes at all; and it's no wonder he's coughing and choking like crazy.

I'm not happy about the prospect of more surgery, but if it will help my son, bring it on. I'm tired of just marking time.

Wednesday, August 19, 2009

Today we went for another CT scan. Since Dylan still needs to be sedated for the test, he will need anesthesia. We have been instructed to actually show up at the adult testing area of the hospital; not sure why, but they must have a reason. We arrive early to the hospital, after another morning of telling my 3 year old he can't eat or drink; and they take him in almost immediately. I help get him changed and comfortable on a stretcher, while the nurses and doctors prep for the test and anesthesia. Once Dylan is sedated, I remind them that he doesn't wake up well from anesthesia, so please let him sleep as long as he can. I am directed to an empty stretcher in the hallway in front of the CT scan room, where I can wait for Dylan. Wow, this is cozy!

After 20 minutes, I hear all sorts of banging and yelling in the room. I look through the window and see Dylan thrashing about and a doctor holding him down. I immediately open the door and ask what is wrong. They say that my son is too violent as he is waking and that someone in this room is going to get hurt. The nurse and anesthesiologist walk out but not before adding a sedative to my son's IV line, which "knocks" him out again. I am standing in this room, alone with Dylan, a 3 year old boy, who was just treated as a zoo animal. The professional staff leaves out of frustration or fear, but the point is that they left. I lay down on the stretcher next to Dylan, not really knowing what to think. I am sad and angry, all at the same time, for how this little child was just treated, especially after I told them what would happen. Another example of how medical professionals really listen to patients.

Shortly after, another nurse comes in and tells me that we are being moved to the Pediatric PACU. Oh, thank goodness! Those nurses know how to take care of kids; and, since we know most of them and are familiar with the area, it was more comfortable for both Dylan and me.

Wednesday, August 26, 2009

The Parade of Doctors continued today with a visit to a cardio-thoracic surgeon, Dr. Kimball. . . . and, to no one's surprise, it will expand even further.

The guy we saw today looked at Dylan's CT scan and delivered some surprising news. He said that Dylan's trachea is crushed because there's a giant blood vessel that's out of place and lying right across it. He can't be sure which specific vessels are causing the problem without further investigation, but he did say that treatment would involve moving major blood vessels and doing a graft in the damaged area of his trachea. Everything after that became a blur of scary terms like bypass machine, respirator, very high risk . . . oh, yeah, and a month or more in the hospital with Dylan in a medically-induced coma for the first two weeks to allow his airway to heal. WHAT????

I was still trying to absorb all of that when he did something no other doctor has done since we started this journey three and a half years ago. He admitted that he couldn't help. He said Dylan's case is too complicated for him.

Wow. At first, I was really disappointed that we'd hit another brick wall. But, after I thought about it, I realized how much I appreciated his honesty. On one hand, we're no closer to an answer; but, on the other hand, at least we're not going to waste time with a doctor who can't help us.

Driving home from the appointment, I couldn't help thinking about how different things might have been if some of the other doctors we've seen – Dr. Barclay (pediatrician) and Dr. Guitano (cardiologist), for example – had just been candid and admitted that either they didn't know what was wrong with Dylan or that the case was beyond their expertise. Whether you're a mom or a teacher or a doctor, there's nothing wrong with admitting that you don't know something. The more I thought about it, the more I appreciated this guy's honesty and his willingness to let us move forward to someone else who might have more experience and expertise.

And, he's going to help us do that. He set up an appointment for us with a Dr. Chapman at a children's medical center in PA. I hate having to go out of town again . . . and I hate even more that he can't see us until October . . . but, at this point, I'll go anywhere and do anything to make my little guy well.

And, yes. I checked to be sure that Dr. Chapman wasn't the same guy we saw in Pennsylvania before – the one who brushed us off in 15 minutes!

Thursday, August 27, 2009

I can't stop thinking about what Dr. Kimball (cardiothoracic) said yesterday, so I dug out my records and re-read everything from the procedure Dylan had in Cleveland – the one we thought would solve all his problems.

Why did no one see this issue with the blood vessels then? They had him opened up and they were RIGHT THERE, looking at his heart and his trachea. It seems like something like that should stick out like a sore thumb. The doctor yesterday certainly had no problem seeing it; but, then again, it was only the radiologist in Hartford who detected the vascular ring in the first place, and no one else believed it was there.

I keep coming back to how one of the nurses in Cleveland kept emphasizing that we should follow up when we got home. She said it several times, and I remember thinking, "Okay. I've got it." I don't know; it just makes me wonder.

Ahh! I can't think about this anymore right now. I just have to figure how where to go from here.

Friday, September 11, 2009

Dylan has been out of pre-school all week, and I don't know when I'll be able to send him back. There's a pretty significant H1N1 outbreak, and I just can't take a chance on letting him contract something so serious. He's sick all the time anyway, but something like that could be fatal for him.

I really, really hate the fact that Dylan isn't able to have the normal childhood that Sydney has. She's rarely sick, but he's always sick. She hardly ever misses school, but he can't go at all. She runs around like crazy; but, when he tries to play like the other kids, he runs out of breath in no time and has to stop. I know he gets frustrated, and so do I. I just want to get this figured out, whatever it takes.

Monday, September 14, 2009

Just came back from our consult with Dr. Russell (Pediatric GI) in Providence. He said the extent of reflux that Dylan is experiencing needs to be assessed and to further evaluate if there are any other stomach/esophagus issues, prior to having surgery. It was explained to me that kids with severe reflux have a higher risk of side effects after surgery and a longer recovery time, due to potential side effects. We don't want that now.

Before I left, an upper endoscopy (which he has had before) and a 24-hour pH monitor test was set up for later this week. I guess they can put in the pH probe while he is under anesthesia for the endoscopy, as to make this process a bit easier on Dylan. Should be a fun week!

Thursday, September 17, 2009

Up bright and early for our drive to Providence to get all this testing underway. Another morning of telling my 3 year old that he can't eat or drink. Ugh! This morning, I decided lambies were NPO, too. It made Dylan feel like he was not suffering alone and redirected his attention away from being hungry and onto keeping a watch over lambies.

So far, the pre-op stuff has gone smoothly; and Dylan was just taken into the OR for the procedure. Lambies and I will rest with some coffee.

Friday, September 18, 2009

What a crazy twenty-four hours! Procedure yesterday was without any hiccup, except for the vomiting all over my mom's car (post anesthesia side effect). His esophagus and stomach looked great (no reflux), despite the large bulge in his esophagus, seemingly caused by where the blood vessel is pushing against it.

The probe thing – well, that was one of my biggest challenges yet. They had placed the tube through Dylan's nose and down his throat into his stomach. It was hooked up to a monitor that he is to wear on him until the whole thing is removed tomorrow. So, when Dylan woke up from anesthesia, what do you think he did first? Yep. He tried to pull the tube out. So, out came the restraints, while I sat on his bed and held his arms down. What a horrible feeling to watch my son be tied down: SCARED because he didn't understand and frustrated because he couldn't relieve the feeling of something in his nose.

We get home and come up with a boat load of distractions to keep his mind off the probe. They sent us home with the restraints, which I had to use initially. Lots of movies and games. I slept with him all night so that he wouldn't wake up and pull it out.

By morning, I was exhausted from the constant struggle. It was all I could do to get Sydney off to school and Dylan to his appointment without pulling the tube out.

Thank goodness, that is over, although he did better than I expected. Forgot - - those results are normal, as well.

Tuesday, September 22, 2009

My head is spinning from trying to get help for this blood-vessel-on-the-trachea thing. I've been on the phone for days with all kinds of experts – Boston Children's Hospital, Miami Children's – just to name two – but no one has an answer.

Still, we've made progress. At least we know what the problem is and that it's vascular rather than an issue with his airway itself. His blood vessels are literally choking him.

But, even though we know what the problem is, no one seems to know how to solve it. Lots of people have guesses about things that might work, but no one has a definitive answer; and I'm not willing to risk my son's life on someone's guess. Our appointment in Pennsylvania is coming soon, so maybe Dr. Chapman will have an idea. He comes highly recommended.

Thursday, October 8, 2009

What an ass! I don't think I've ever met a man as arrogant as the great Dr. Chapman. I'm so angry and frustrated, I could just scream.

We flew to Pennsylvania for our long-awaited appointment. We arrived a few minutes early, and I'd brought a lot of books and toys for Dylan because I expected that we'd be there for a while. I'm a veteran of these introductory appointments by now, and they usually take a long time because there's so much to discuss with a case as complicated as Dylan's.

I couldn't have been more wrong. It was déjà vu from our trip to PA a couple of years ago. We were in and out in 15 minutes – AGAIN – and when we left, it was a struggle to keep Dylan from seeing how upset I was.

First, the guy was completely unprepared. He wasn't familiar with any of Dylan's mountain of test results that had been forwarded to him; and, in fact, he said he'd have to repeat all of them. How ridiculous is that? Dylan has had every test in the book, and the results are all RIGHT THERE; but Dr. Chapman was insistent that we'd have to repeat everything, including the CT scan from just a few weeks ago. Those things involve an enormous amount of radiation, and I'm not about to put Dylan through that risk, unless it's absolutely necessary.

While I was still trying to absorb that demand, Dr. Chapman proceeded to describe what he proposed to do. He wanted to remove the descending aorta and use a plastic graft to close off that side of Dylan's aortic arch, which I guess makes sense; but then he said he'd have to repeat the procedure every three or four years as Dylan continues to grow.

That's not the worst of it, though. He went on at length about the high risk of fatality with this surgery, and he said – right in front of Dylan – that he could very likely die. I was stunned. This kid isn't an infant anymore. He's a bright, attentive almost-four-year-old who understands everything. What kind of doctor says something like that in front of a child???

Needless to say, I'm not going to let this pompous idiot anywhere near my son with a scalpel, unless I've exhausted every other possibility. What a waste of time and money, although Dylan did enjoy the plane ride!

Two strikes against Pennsylvania doctors now. I don't think we'll give them a third opportunity.

Thursday, November 5, 2009

I have a new ally. It turns out that my sister-in-law Susan has a friend whose husband is a cardiovascular surgeon, and she offered to ask him to review Dylan's case and see if he has any suggestions. I made a copy of all of Dylan's records (which could fill a library by now) and sent them to this doctor, so we'll see if he has any new ideas. His name is Emmett Dean McKenzie, and he's at Texas Children's Hospital in Houston – not exactly in the neighborhood – but I'm tired of spinning my wheels while my little boy continues to suffer. If he can help, I'll start packing our bags for Houston.

Tuesday, November 10, 2009

Susan is my new hero! Dr. McKenzie went over all of Dylan's history (unlike others who have barely glanced at his records), and he called me directly and spent an hour on the phone with me. AN HOUR! He explained what the problem is and how to fix it PERMANENTLY.

First of all, he was very knowledgeable about Dylan's condition. He's got extensive experience and – here's the best part – he's even developed a new procedure that he says corrects the problem the first time. No one has offered anything like that before. Even the doctors who think they have some sort of solution say he'd need more surgeries as he grows, but Dr. McKenzie is very confident that his procedure would eliminate the need for that.

He explained that he would disconnect the descending aorta right after the arch and move it to the opposite side of the trachea and esophagus, then connect it into the ascending aorta. Then, he'd seal off the open end of the arch, using Dylan's own tissue; and that would relieve the pressure. And, because he'd use Dylan's tissue rather than plastic to make the repair, the tissue would just grow right along with him. He says he's had a lot of success and after reviewing Dylan's case thinks he's an excellent candidate.

Even though it's a serious surgery, the risk is low. This guy was so calm and reassuring, and he spoke in a way that I could understand everything he told me. He explained everything in great detail and answered all my questions (unlike that jackass in Philadelphia). His confidence gives me confidence.

Going all the way to Texas isn't my first choice, obviously; but, apparently, we'll just have to make one trip. Dr. McKenzie said we don't have to do a preliminary visit for tests – just arrive a few days before the procedure, and they'll do all the pre-op stuff then.

So . . . after our hour-long conversation, we scheduled the surgery. I thought I'd be nervous about it, but I feel nothing but confidence in this doctor. He really seems to know what he's doing, and I'm ready to leap. We set the date for January 13, 2010. Maybe we'll finally have a happy New Year.

Sunday, November 29, 2009

I spent some time on the computer today setting up our "CarePage" for Dylan's surgery. It's a pretty inspired concept. The hospital in Houston hooked us up with an organization that helps kids' parents set up a website and message board, so we can keep people at home updated about Dylan's surgery and recuperation; and friends and family members can post messages to us as we go along.

I got it set up tonight with the information about the date of Dylan's procedure. Now, all I have to do is share the link with anybody we want to keep updated. I hope I'll have time to keep up with it while we're in Houston. On the other hand, maybe it will help me fill the time I'm sure to spend waiting around the hospital.

Thursday, December 3, 2009

Dylan is now what my grandmother would call a "shut in!" We have to be super careful to avoid exposing him to anything that could compromise his surgery next month; and, of course, germs are everywhere this time of year.

To be as cautious as possible, Dr. McKenzie has put Dylan on social interaction restrictions – no school, no public places, and no large parties, nothing that would bring him into contact with anything that could make him sick. It's going to be hard, especially with his birthday and the holidays coming up; but we've come too far to take chances now. Everything is set, so I don't want to have to postpone this any longer.

Wednesday, December 9, 2009

My little guy is four years old today! And, what a wild four years it has been! – nothing like I'd expected when I was in the hospital giving birth to him. It's been tough, to say the least, but I wouldn't trade my Dylan for the healthiest kid in the world. He faces all his challenges with such courage. I really admire him.

We had a low-key celebration at home. If this surgery is successful, maybe next year we'll have a blow-out party somewhere special!

Thursday, December 24, 2009

Christmas Eve already! Things were a bit different for us this year, with Dylan's pre-surgery restrictions. We'd already skipped all the usual holiday parties; and tonight we didn't even go to Mom's house for the annual family dinner. I missed seeing everyone and felt a little lonely tonight, but it will be worth it if we can keep Dylan strong and healthy until time for his surgery.

Saturday, January 9, 2010

We're in Texas! The past few weeks have gone by in a blur. The holidays were low-key. There has been so much to do to get ready for this trip; and, either Mike or I have had to be at home with Dylan all the time, since he couldn't go out.

After a lot of thought, we decided to bring the whole family here for the weekend. I wanted everyone, but especially Sydney, to see where Dylan will be and be able to picture us during these next few days. Sydney doesn't talk much about it, but I can tell she's really worried about her little brother. Rather than trying to explain the whole procedure, we've told both Sydney and Dylan that we're here because we've finally found a doctor who can operate on Dylan and fix his cough. That seems to be enough for now, but Sydney is still concerned. Dylan has only had one question – "How many shots am I going to get?" I can't very well say, "Shots are the least of it, honey!"

This place is truly the definition of a medical center. There is something like thirty hospitals in the couple of blocks around our hotel, so it's going to take us a little time to find our way around. I think we'll spend most of the day tomorrow getting acquainted with the area and doing some sightseeing before most of the family goes home on Monday. Houston has a nice aquarium that the kids want to see, so we'll probably hit that.

Monday, January 11, 2010

Busy day! We had to say goodbye to Mike, Liam, Sydney, and my father. They headed back to Connecticut for work and school, but Mom stayed with Dylan and me. I don't know what I'd do without her support.

The rest of the day was a whirlwind of pre-op testing in the morning. At 3:00 p.m., we had our first face-to-face consultation with Dr. McKenzie. He was everything I'd hoped for and more! Just as he had been on the phone, he was so reassuring. He encouraged me to ask all the questions I wanted, and he was great about explaining everything that would happen and what we could expect in the next few days. He was great with Dylan, too, which I loved. Even though he's only four, I think it's important for him to like the doctor who's about to operate on him; and I think he really did.

I feel so good tonight. A little nervous, but so encouraged by the hospital staff and, especially, Dr. McKenzie. I'm glad we're here.

Tuesday, January 12, 2010

Another exhausting day. Seven hours of pre-op testing. There can't be much they don't know about Dylan by this time, but I'm glad they're so thorough. My confidence in these people is continuing to increase.

BUT, we had an "incident" this afternoon. We were in an exam room waiting for the next test – I forget which one – and Dylan fell off the exam table and landed on his head! After all the precautions we've taken to keep him healthy for the surgery, I couldn't believe it. We've avoided every germ and now they're worried that he might have a concussion!

I hope hope hope they don't have to postpone the surgery because of this. I'm geared up for it now. I think Dylan is, too; so I just want to move forward at this point.

Wednesday, January 13, 2010

Surgery Day! We got up early because we had to be ready at 7:00 a.m. Dylan looked so small but completely adorable in his little hospital gown! He was such a good patient and didn't seem nervous or upset at all. He's just looking forward to having his cough fixed. Mom was a little nervous; but she didn't let him see that, which was good.

They took him to the OR at about 8:00 a.m., leaving us and his lambies to stew for what they said could be a five to eight-hour procedure. I spent a lot of time keeping people updated on our CarePage, as we received information, and just trying to keep myself occupied.

Having Dylan's father in the waiting room with us added to my stress. Our relationship is tense at this point, over visitation and medication issues and the lack of civil communication, in general.

During surgery, the first thing they did was check Dylan's airway to see how much damage there actually was. Someone came out at about 10:30 a.m. to tell us that the airway was severely compressed but that the extent of damage was undeterminable until after the aortic relocation had occurred. That would determine if they needed to reconstruct the trachea or not, so we went back to waiting and hoping.

We got another update around 1:00 p.m., saying that Dylan was on the heart-lung machine and that the real work had started. A little before 3:00 p.m., we learned that Dr. McKenzie had successfully moved the aorta and reconnected it in a new spot; and they'd started the process of returning his blood to normal circulation. That was a bit of a tense time for me. On one hand, it was such a relief to know that the bulk of the work had been done and everything had gone well; but, if his blood didn't circulate properly with the new configuration, we wouldn't be any better off than we'd been originally. He could have had even more problems. But, a little while later, they came back out to say that everything looked great. What a relief! So grateful for all the prayers.

By 6:00 p.m., the procedure was over. Dylan was in recovery, and Dr. McKenzie came out to talk to me. He said the airway had been more compressed than he'd expected but that it recovered really well after the aorta was moved and the pressure was off. He also found a small hole in Dylan's heart and repaired that. The pressure from his aorta had caused quite a bit of damage to his esophagus, but that should start to improve now; and he should have an easier time eating and drinking.

After he got to the ICU, apparently Dylan was crying for me, so I was called in to try to calm him down. WOW! I was surprised that he was already awake and pretty alert. Then, he started asking for food and water, so that's got to be a good sign! He's been such a brave little man, and I'm so proud of him. They're going to keep his blood pressure low overnight to give his new insides a chance to heal, but he's breathing well and isn't complaining at all.

I'm a very grateful person tonight. I'm grateful to Mom for being such a rock today. I'm grateful to Mike and the rest of our family for all their support and to the many, many friends who followed our CarePage and posted messages of support and prayer all day while we waited. I'm grateful to Dylan for being such a courageous little guy and, most of all, I'm grateful to Dr. McKenzie and his amazing staff here at the hospital. Dylan – and the rest of us – couldn't have been in better hands.

Sitting there looking at Dylan tonight, I couldn't help but think that things are going to be very different from now on. As soon as we get home, I'm going to have to start a serious exercise routine and increase my coffee consumption considerably. When this kid is all healed, I think I'll have a very different little boy on my hands!

Thursday, January 14, 2010

First post-op day, and the little guy is improving steadily. He did really well overnight. The first thing this morning he asked for some
hot chocolate, orange juice, a cookie and, of course, his lambies. He
got ice chips and apple juice instead, but he was okay with that! He
also wanted to know when he could see Sydney, which I thought was
very sweet. He loves his big sister. By early morning, his white blood
count was back down – close to normal – as it had skyrocketed last
night, which was worrisome. He hadn't developed a fever, so that
was good news.

Before noon, they had removed three of his six connections, so that
made him more comfortable. I think the tape removal process hurt
worse than the actual surgery. He was happy when THAT was done.
Throughout the day, he was able to eat and drink a bit – just a few
bites of food and some juice; but he's getting it down with no problems. Around mid-day, they got him onto his feet long enough to
move him into a bigger, more comfortable bed; and later we moved
into a room on the cardiac unit.

Most of the day was spent just trying to keep him comfortable. He
did pick up a bit of a cough, so they're trying to get his lungs inflated
a little more to get rid of that. So far, so good. The staff is more than
impressed with how well he's doing.

Me? I fueled up on Starbucks all day. We'll see how much sleep I get
tonight. I'm tired but also on a bit of a high because things are going
so well.

Friday, January 15, 2010

After another good night, Dylan is starting to eat more; and they've taken him off fluid restrictions, so he can drink whatever he wants now. He still has the chest tube – not sure when that will be removed; but he doesn't complain about it. He was able to get out of bed today and even take a lap around the floor. He's still weak, obviously. He spent most of the day just hanging out and watching cartoons with lambies. I also read him the messages that people have continued to leave on the CarePage, and he seemed happy that so many people knew he'd had surgery and were thinking about him.

Saturday, January 16, 2010

I can't believe it, but it looks like Dylan might be discharged tomorrow!

He had a good night and another great day. They took out the chest tube late in the afternoon, and all his tests came back great. It's amazing how quickly children recover, even from major trauma to their bodies. He continues to impress the hospital staff (and his mom!). It seems like such a miracle. I know he's got a long recovery process ahead, but I feel optimistic about his future for the first time in a long, long time.

Sunday, January 17, 2010

We're out! Dylan was discharged today, and we went to Susan and Patrick's house (in Houston), where we all got settled in. They're so great to give us a place to stay for a few days while Dylan continues with his recovery. We'll see Dr. McKenzie on Wednesday, and then it looks like we'll be able to go home over the weekend. I'm so excited to see Mike, Sydney, and Liam again; and so is Dylan.

Monday, January 18, 2010

As happy as Dylan is to be out of the hospital, he realized today that he's not quite well and still has some distance to cover before he really feels good. All the activity yesterday – getting out of the hospital, driving here to Susan and Patrick's, getting settled and so on – involved a lot more moving around than he'd done in the hospital, even with regular walks; so he's pretty sore today. He lay low most of the day and just rested. Hopefully, he'll feel better tomorrow. He needs to get rested for his check-up with Dr. McKenzie and then the trip home. HOME! Can't wait to sleep in my own bed.

While Dylan was napping, I went through my datebook from last year to transfer the birthdays to this year's book; and I started counting the number of medical appointments Dylan has had. I knew it was a lot, but the actual number still shocked me – 58!!!!!!! That includes check-ups, tests, surgeries, and outpatient procedures – the whole circus. If he's had that many in a year, imagine how many there have been in all the years since we started on this merry-go-round.

Tuesday, January 19, 2010

Since we are staying with two doctors, I felt comfortable taking an hour break to get out of the house for a bit. Susan and Patrick have been great about taking care of us, so I thought I'd help out a bit by bringing home dinner. I got Jell-o, chips, and fruit for Dylan and grinders for the rest of us.

I got back to the house, and we put everything out on the table. Then, the most miraculous thing happened. Dylan grabbed a grinder and proceeded to eat the whole thing! He's never eaten a sandwich before because his esophagus has been so constricted that it just wasn't possible to get something like that down his throat. But, there he was, chewing and swallowing that huge grinder just like any other hungry kid. Not only did that make me realize how much better he was feeling but, for the first time, I really began to get a sense of how different his life is going to be. Well – how different ALL our lives are going to be.

I had such high hopes for this surgery, and I was pretty optimistic about the outcome but, holy cow! I never dreamed Dylan would get so much better so fast. Of course, I had no dinner; but, hey! I can't begrudge him a grinder. The kid has a lot of eating to catch up on.

Wednesday, January 20, 2010

We've cleared the last hurdle, and we're ready to go home! Saw Dr. McKenzie today, and he said Dylan is doing GREAT. It looks like the surgery was very successful. He's recovering normally, maybe even a little ahead of schedule. Obviously, we need to check in with his regular doctors back in Connecticut next week. They've been staying in touch and are so happy that we've apparently gotten this resolved after all the starts and stops of the past four years.

I'm still pretty bitter about some of the incompetence; but, right now, it's hard for me to feel anything but happy. We're not completely out of the woods. Dylan will have a good six to eight weeks of recovery, and we'll still have to restrict his activities and avoid public places until he's completely healed. And, it's too soon to tell what the future holds for him. There might be permanent damage to his airway and esophagus. He might have scarring or other issues with his lungs. He might be more susceptible to illness or have more difficulty fighting it off than other people do. There are a million things that could go wrong, but there are also a lot of things than could go right; and that's enough for me right now.

I've been doing a lot of reflecting over the past few days, thinking back to everything we've been through since Dylan was born that snowy night more than four years ago. The thing I keep coming back to is this. I wish I could talk to other moms who suspect that something might be wrong with their child but can't get a doctor to listen or act. I'd tell them to trust their instincts. From the time Dylan was just a few days old, I knew in my heart that something wasn't right, but so many doctors insinuated – or even told me outright – that it was all in my head and that I was just an over-anxious new mother. I'm so glad I didn't listen to them and ignore my instincts. I really can't bear to think about what my son's future might have been if I hadn't been persistent and fought for him. It was frustrating and lonely, but so worth it in the end.

And now, I have to start getting our things packed. I'm heading back to Connecticut with a little guy who will soon be leading the life of a typical four-year-old boy. Look out, world!

Addendum

As of today, Dylan is a healthy 7-year-old boy, who loves to run, climb, and play. He has been involved with soccer and karate and loves to swim. Though the struggles of his early years are behind us, there are a few residual effects that are evaluated in checkups with Cardiology, Pulmonology, and GI. It seems that Dylan's esophagus might have some nerve damage, caused from the aorta pushing against the esophagus. This seems to have disrupted the normal flow of food through the esophagus to the stomach, resulting in aspiration to the lungs. This is what has caused all those tests to show high levels of inflammation in his lungs, resulting in scaring. With a small amount of medication, the issue at hand seems to be controlled. This diagnosis and treatment plan comes from another out-of-box thinker, Dylan's newest G.I. doctor, from Norwalk, CT. For the moment, we have accepted these potential side effects with ease, as the issues that used to be at the forefront of our daily existence are almost a mere memory.

If You Think a Loved-One Is Sick

I have a Master's Degree in nursing, yet I struggled for four years to find out what was wrong with my son and get him the help he needed. Even with my education and experience, it was very difficult to get anyone to listen to me; so I can only imagine how frustrating it must be for those without a medical background to navigate the quagmire that our health care system has become. It's common to feel powerless, but the fact is that we do have power; and we shouldn't be afraid to use it.

- If you feel that your child or another loved one is ill, there are steps you can take.
- Trust your instincts! If you think something is wrong, it probably is.
- Don't rely on your primary care physician alone. He or she is your first resource; but you might need to seek the help of specialists, perhaps even specialists in several different areas. Get as many opinions as it takes.
- Don't assume that if a case is too complicated your doctor will direct you to another practitioner who is better qualified. Ask for a referral, if you think one is warranted; and push until you get it.
- Don't be intimidated by your doctors or other health care professionals. Physicians should be respected for their knowledge and expertise; but they are not gods, and they are fallible.
- Look for help from a variety of sources. Reach out to anyone who might know someone in the health care field and can provide a contact. I would never have found Dr. McKenzie without the help of my sister-in-law.
- Ask questions – a lot of them. Before an appointment, take

time to write down your questions. Take notes when your doctor answers them, so you can review the information later. And, if your doctor doesn't take enough time to answer your questions, change doctors.

- Always get a copy of your test results before you leave the office, lab or hospital. You are entitled to have a copy of any and all tests, including a CD of CT scans, MRIs, x-rays, mammograms, etc. Even if you can't read them yourself, you might need to show them to other experts in the future.
- Keep thorough, meticulous records. You never know when you might need them, and your memory fades as time passes.
- Most important, don't give up – ever. The answer is out there somewhere, so keep fighting for your loved one until you find it.
- Oh, and by the way….we couldn't have done it without his guardian angels, the lambies! Clearly, a Higher Power knew one was not enough.

About a Vascular Ring

Vascular ring is an abnormal formation of the aorta, the large artery that carries blood from the heart to the rest of the body. It is a congenital problem, which means it is present at birth. In fact, it occurs very early in the baby's development in the womb.

Vascular ring is rare, accounting for less than one per cent of all congenital heart problems. It occurs as often in males as females, and some infants who have a vascular ring also have other congenital heart problems.

Normally, the aorta develops from one of several curved pieces of tissue called arches. The body breaks down some of the remaining arches, while others form into arteries. Some arches that should break down do not, and they are still present when the baby is born. These arches form a ring of blood vessels that press down on the trachea and esophagus.

There are several types of vascular rings, including a double aortic arch, which is the type Dylan had. In most cases, symptoms are seen during infancy; and these typically include a high-pitched or barking cough, loud breathing, frequent pneumonia or respiratory infections, respiratory distress, and wheezing. In addition to breathing issues, pressure on the trachea and esophagus can also lead to digestive problems. Digestive symptoms are less common but might include choking, difficulty eating solid foods, difficulty swallowing, GERD, slow breast or bottle feeding, and vomiting. The more pressure the ring exerts, the more severe the symptoms will be.

When a child's vascular ring produces symptoms, surgery is usually performed as soon as possible to split the ring and relieve the pressure on the surrounding structures. Delaying surgery can lead to serious complications, including damage to the trachea and even death. Those who do not have symptoms might not need treatment, but they should be watched carefully in case the condition worsens.

Referenced from: A.D.A.M. Medical Encyclopedia. Atlanta (GA): A.D.A.M.; 2011.

Acknowledgements

I am forever grateful to all those who truly made a difference in Dylan's life: from the nurses in the frequently visited PACU to the radiology staff in more than eleven facilities; to the Child Life Specialists and Toy Cart Donors; and to all the friends and family that supported us in more ways than I can mention.

Very special thanks to Carrie Sartor who not only took care of Dylan during the toughest years of his life but left an everlasting mark on our family.

And finally, I am forever indebted to Texas Children's Hospital, Houston. Without the professional expertise and compassionate care provided by the entire staff, especially Dr. Emmett Dean McKenzie, this book might have had a different ending. I would also like to thank Dr. Regina Palazzo, Dr. David Karas, Dr. Peter Dixon and all of their staff for scheduling, faxing, and coordinating everything over the last six years and, most of all, for their compassion and out-of-the-box thinking.

Parade of Doctors

* Dr. Matteo and

* Dr. Colbert: Pediatrics - #1

* Dr. Barclay: Pediatrics - #2

* Dr. Feinstein: Ear, Nose & Throat - #1

* Dr. Boyer: Gastroenterology - #1 (New Haven)

* Dr. Guitano: Cardiology (New Haven)

* Dr. Hallisey: Gastroenterology - #2 (Hartford)

* Dr. Henzin: Cardiothoracic Surgery - #1 (Cleveland)

* Dr. Bosco: Cardiothoracic Surgery - #2 (Boston)

* Dr. Penn: Cardiothoracic Surgery - #3 (PA consult #1)

  Dr. Karas: Ear, Nose & Throat – #2 (New Haven)

* Dr. Bennett: Pulmonology - #1 (Hartford)

  Dr. Palazzo: Pulmonology - #2 (New Haven)

* Dr. Kimball: Cardiothoracic Surgery - #4 (New Haven)

* Dr. Russell: Gastroenterology - #3 (Providence, RI)

* Dr. Chapman: Cardiothoracic Surgery - #5 (PA consult #2)

  Dr. McKenzie: Cardiothoracic Surgery - #6 (Houston)

* The names of these doctors have been changed, due to the sensitive nature of this story.

www.ingramcontent.com/pod-product-compliance
Lightning Source LLC
LaVergne TN
LVHW021458080426
835509LV00018B/2329